Computers in Clinical Practice

Also Available from the American College of Physicians

American College of Physicians Home Care Guide for Cancer

Clinical Practice Guidelines, 1995 Edition

Common Diagnostic Tests: Use and Interpretation–Second Edition

Common Screening Tests

Diagnostic Strategies for Common Medical Problems

Drug Prescribing in Renal Failure: Dosing Guidelines for Adults–Third Edition

Guide for Adult Immunization–Third Edition

International Medical Graduates in U.S. Hospitals: A Guide for Program Directors and Applicants

Learning from Practitioners: Office-Based Teaching of Internal Medicine Residents

On Being a Doctor

Software for Internists: Critical Evaluations from *Medical Software Reviews* and the Journal Literature

This is Our Work: The Legacy of Sir William Osler

Publications from the *British Medical Journal* are distributed in North America by the American College of Physicians.

Our *Resources for Internists* catalog and ordering information for the American College of Physicians, *British Medical Journal* publications, and ACP Product Discount Service products are available from:

Customer Service Center
American College of Physicians
Independence Mall West
Sixth Street at Race
Philadelphia, PA 19106-1572
215-351-2600
800-523-1546, ext. 2600

Note on Products Mentioned (and Not Mentioned) in This Book

The purpose of this book is to introduce readers to the types of information resources currently available and to describe how these resources can support information management in clinical practice. It is not the intent of the editor or publisher to provide either a complete listing of useful available products or a formal evaluation of specific resources; therefore, the inclusion (or exclusion) of a specific product should not be viewed as an endorsement (or nonendorsement) of that product.

Continuing Medical Education Credit for Reading This Book

Outside of business settings, information technology applications are frequently viewed as entertainment, productivity, or general education tools. A key premise of this book is that clinical computing tools can be a valuable ingredient in the practitioner's delivery of optimal patient care. As such, the time you invest learning about these tools by reading *Computers in Clinical Practice* is an important component of your continuing professional development. We encourage you to consider recording and reporting (where acceptable) the time you spend reading this book as part of your continuing medical education (CME) activities. For example, you may claim up to 30 hours of Category 2 credit for self-directed learning (that is, activities such as literature reading that are not administered by an accredited organization) toward the American Medical Association Physician Recognition Award (AMA-PRA). You should check the applicable rules with the organization (for example, state medical society) to whom you will be reporting these credits.

Computers in Clinical Practice

Managing Patients, Information, and Communication

Edited by Jerome A. Osheroff, MD

American College of Physicians
Philadelphia, Pennsylvania

The ACP Information Technology Series

Printed in the United States of America.

Library of Congress Cataloging-in-Publication Data

Computers in clinical practice: managing patients, information, and
   communication / edited by Jerome A. Osheroff.
        p.   cm.— (The ACP information technology series)
   Includes index.
   ISBN 0-943126-33-9 : $45.00 (est.) $35.00 (est.) to members
   1. Medical informatics. 2. Medical offices—Automation.
3. Medicine—Data processing. I. Osheroff, Jerome A., 1959–
II. Series.
   [DNLM: 1. Medical Informatics. 2. Medical Records Systems,
Computerized. 3. Diagnosis, Computer-Assisted. 4. Therapy,
Computer-Assisted. 5. Patient Education. W 26.5 C7388 1995]
R858.C65375 1995
610'.285—dc20
DNLM/DLC
for Library of Congress   95-7875
                                          CIP

Library of Congress Catalog Card No. 95-7875

ISBN 0-943126-33-9

CONTRIBUTORS

Lawrence Blonde, MD, FACP
Vice-Chair, Department of Medicine
Ochsner Clinic and
The Alton Ochsner Medical Foundation
New Orleans, Louisiana

Barry H. Blumenfeld, MD, MS
Director of Product Development
First DataBank
San Bruno, California

Jerome H. Carter, MD, FACP
Assistant Professor of Medicine
Division of General Internal Medicine
University of Alabama—Birmingham
Birmingham, Alabama

Matthew Cushing, MD, FACP
Mill Valley Medical Group
Mill Valley, California

William M. Detmer, MD, FACP
Assistant Clinical Professor of Medicine
University of California, San Francisco
San Francisco, California

Paul N. Gorman, MD, FACP
Assistant Professor of Medicine and
  Health Informatics
Biomedical Information
  Communications Center
Oregon Health Science University
Portland, Oregon

Richard D. Guthrie, Jr., MD
Ochsner Clinic
New Orleans, Louisiana

Robert Hayward, MD
Assistant Professor
Health Information Research Unit
McMaster University Health Science Centre
Hamilton, Ontario, Canada

Edward P. Hoffer, MD, FACP
Assistant Director
Laboratory of Computer Science
Massachusetts General Hospital
Boston, Massachusetts

Gary Kahn, MD, MEd
Assistant Clinical Professor
Department of Preventive Medicine
  and Biometry
Medical Information Sector
University of Colorado School of Medicine
Boulder, Colorado

Paul Kleeberg, MD
St. Peter Clinic
St. Peter, Minnesota

Daniel R. Masys, MD, FACP
Director of Biomedical Informatics
School of Medicine
University of California, San Diego
La Jolla, California

Clement J. McDonald, MD, FACP
Distinguished Professor of Medicine
Indiana University School of Medicine
Indianapolis, Indiana

K. Ann McKibbon, MLS
Research Coordinator
Clinical Epidemiology and Biostatistics
McMaster University Health Science Centre
Hamilton, Ontario, Canada

Blackford Middleton, MD, FACP
Medical Director, Information Management
  and Technology
Stanford Health Services
Stanford, California

Mark A. Musen, MD, PhD, FACP
Head, Section on Medical Informatics
Stanford University School of Medicine
Stanford, California

Jerome A. Osheroff, MD, FACP
American College of Physicians and
Adjunct Assistant Professor of Medicine
University of Pennsylvania
Philadelphia, Pennsylvania

Marc Overhage, MD, PhD
Associate Professor of Medicine
Indiana University School of Medicine
Indianapolis, Indiana

Karin Rex
Owner
ComputerEase
North Wales, Pennsylvania

Donald L. Vine, MD, FACP
Associate Professor of Medicine
University of Kansas School of Medicine
Wichita, Kansas

Michael H. Zaroukian, MD, PhD, FACP
Associate Professor of Medicine
Michigan State University
East Lansing, Michigan

REVIEWERS

The editor wishes to express his thanks to the following peer reviewers for reading draft chapters from this publication and offering many helpful suggestions on the content and presentation of the material.

Alan Aronson, MD, FACP

H. Verdain Barnes, MD, FACP

Lettia Carlson, MD

Jeffrey Carstens, MD, USN

David B. Case, MD, FACP

Frank Davidoff, MD, FACP

Daniel C. Davis, MD, FACP

Donald Deye, MD

F. Daniel Duffy, MD, FACP

Marc D. Grobman, DO

William R. Hersh, MD, FACP

Edward P. Hoffer, MD, FACP

David C. Hurwitz, MD

Robert J. Kapicka, MD

Raphael J. Kiel, MD, FACP

David J. Kumaki, MD, FACP

Steven E. Labkoff, MD

Scott C. Litin, MD, FACP

Frank W. Meissner, MD, FACP

Stuart J. Nelson, MD, FACP

Howard H. Schubiner, MD, FACP

Bruce Slater, MD

Robert S. Spena, DSW

Christopher D. Wilhelm, MD, FACP

Contents

FOREWORD

The governance and staff of the American College of Physicians (ACP) are committed to ensuring that ACP plays a vital role in providing education and information to clinical practitioners. We believe that computer-based technologies will continue to be increasingly valuable for providing access to information, communication, and education in the rapidly changing and information-rich health care environment. Accordingly, we are developing a broad array of products and services designed to help clinicians understand and make optimal use of these new information management tools. This book is a milestone in that effort.

The College has recognized for some time the importance of using computer-based technologies to support physicians' activities. In 1981, ACP created the Telecommunications Subcommittee of the Education Policy Committee to consider this issue; that subcommittee's mission was "to examine areas where ACP can become involved in the application of computers in medicine"—a simple mission statement for a complex issue. Over the years, the College's focus on this topic has evolved and intensified. The results of this evolution are manifest in the increasing variety of information technology-related education programs and information management products offered by ACP. An overview of these offerings can be found at the beginning of the Appendix.

While we are proud of these programs, we believe that much more needs to be done to ensure that useful information technology applications are developed and used appropriately. The next phase of evolution of clinical information resources and services should be marked by a much closer collaboration between product and program developers and users than has taken place in the past. We would like to help create a tighter partnership between the College and users of information technology, and we hope that developers and vendors can be brought into this process as well.

To begin the process, I invite you to contact me with your comments on ACP's activities and role in this area. How well are we meeting your needs for support in managing clinical information? What can we do that is new or different to meet your needs better? As our projects and plans evolve, we intend to share them with you via online channels such as ACP Online and printed channels such as *ACP Observer*. We invite you to share your experiences using new information resources in practice with us and with your colleagues via these same channels.

We anticipate that *Computers in Clinical Practice* will answer many questions but also generate many more. Your input helps to ensure that our offerings best meet your ongoing needs. I look forward to hearing any questions or comments you have about the use of computers in medicine or about the College's programs in this area.

Robert Spena, DSW
American College of Physicians
Telephone: 215-351-2570; Fax: 215-351-2594
CompuServe: 75300,633
Internet: bobsp@acp.mhs.compuserve.com

Editor's Acknowledgments

Many people at the American College of Physicians have contributed to this project, but several deserve special mention. Kathy Case and Bob Spena recognized early the importance of the publication and provided the push for it to develop; Bob provided special support, input, and guidance throughout the project. Pamela Fried offered her patience and professionalism in directing the publication to fruition, while Frank Davidoff lent his support to the project in general and gave helpful input on two of the chapters in particular. Diane McCabe, Gina Jones, and Jeanine Casler are acknowledged for their administrative and editorial contributions, and Mike Ripca is acknowledged for his graphic and design assistance. The College's Medical Informatics Subcommittee also deserves special mention for its continued support and input; each of the seven members has served as either a chapter author or a peer reviewer.

Many others outside the College staff also deserve special acknowledgment. I am indebted to Bob Manning for his work on an earlier version of this book and to each of the chapter authors for the experience and insight they skillfully brought to bear in addressing the central questions of each chapter. I am grateful to Peter Dorman for his role in enhancing the structure and presentation of all the material on these pages and even more grateful to him for the help he has given me in maturing as a writer and editor. Thanks to Peter also for contributing the Glossary. I would also like to thank Pat Wieland for her attention to detail and her editorial support throughout this project. Similarly, I am indebted to my many clinical and informatics colleagues whose guidance has helped me to productively focus on improving patient care through better information management. And many thanks go out to those individuals dispersed throughout cyberspace who responded to my electronic-mail queries during the development of this book; their ability to participate meaningfully and efficiently in the process is another confirmation of the power of the digital information age.

Finally, I would like to express my appreciation to my family for their important contributions to this effort: to my wife Patty for helping me deliver the very best I can in all I do; to my young sons Zachary and Jason for their patience and continued interest in the project during the long nights and weekends that this book occupied much of my attention; and to my parents, siblings, and extended family for their inexhaustible support and encouragement.

Jerome A. Osheroff, MD, FACP
CompuServe: 72262,2323
Internet: jerryo@acp.mhs.compuserve.com

INTRODUCTION
IMPROVING CLINICAL INFORMATION MANAGEMENT IN EVERYDAY MEDICAL PRACTICE

Jerome A. Osheroff, MD, FACP

. . . .

Caring for patients is a wonderful privilege and responsibility, but providing the most efficient and effective care requires clinicians to retain or have easy access to large amounts of medical information. The volume and complexity of medical knowledge and data today have far outstripped any physician's ability to function optimally without the support of information management tools. Yet many physicians are uncertain how to implement these tools in their daily medical activities.

The Purpose of This Book

The goal of this book is threefold: to help you understand how your practice can benefit from modern information technology; to familiarize you with the wide variety of software available for the many areas of your professional activity; and to help you implement these technologies in your practice when you are ready.

Imagine practicing medicine in an environment where there are no obstacles to accessing or exchanging information exactly when, where, and in the form it is needed. Imagine how rewarding it would be to have the following capabilities and supports:

- A practice management system that optimally supports the business components of your practice

- Access to just the right information about your patients wherever you are, whenever you need it

- Patient problem and medication lists that are readily available before each patient visit and easily updated during the visit

- Automatic checking of drug interactions and printing of prescriptions and instructions at the end of each visit

- Programs to make teaching patients even more enjoyable, effective, and efficient

- Instantaneous, fingertip access to an authoritative, convenient-to-use guideline or other reference on a problematic clinical issue

- Decision support tools for diagnosis and therapy that conveniently supply missing information necessary for making the most up-to-date, accurate, and efficient clinical decisions

- Ready access to thousands of colleagues with a vast collective expertise for curbside consults

- Convenient, cost-effective, enjoyable, and useful products for supporting your continued professional education and development.

While the existence of computer-based resources will not automatically bring about this clinical utopia, modern information technology will play an increasingly important role in making this vision a reality.

Information technology can make it easier to perform functions such as accessing current information; doing repetitive or time-consuming tasks (for example, generating prescriptions and maintaining a schedule for patient visits); and communicating conveniently with many geographically dispersed colleagues. From a broader perspective, claims have been made that the various clinical information management products can improve patient outcomes, increase your satisfaction with your practice, and improve the efficiency and effectiveness of your practice and enhance its revenue. Evidence in support of these claims, however, is primarily anecdotal.

Right now you can buy computer-based tools that

approximate to varying degrees the information-processing functions for the capabilities listed above. Despite the significant utility of these resources, they do not yet optimally satisfy the information management needs of clinical practice. Major barriers exist to smoothly integrating these resources into the daily work flow and fully using their potential. In addition, there is significant room for improving these products. Clinical application of information technology is so complex, broad, and new that practical overviews on this topic are difficult to find.

We who have worked on this book hope that it serves all those interested in applying computer-based resources to the management of clinical information. For those unfamiliar with information technology, we have tried to make the material easily understandable and practical. Even though a growing number of physicians are becoming comfortable using computers, and some are already using clinical software, most clinicians have not yet begun to fully utilize the powerful clinical resources currently available. The technologic breadth covered in this guide is such that even sophisticated users of clinical computing resources should find new and useful information.

Practitioners, whether established or just starting out, should use this book to learn how the technology can help them and how to make the best use of available products. Administrators or practitioners responsible for introducing clinical information management technology to their group or institution should also find this book useful. And we hope those who teach residents, medical students, and others about the clinical uses of information technology will find this guide valuable. We expect, moreover, that this book will inspire researchers, product developers, and others to add better and more integrated clinical information tools to those now available.

The State of the Art in Medical Information Technology

When asked about the components necessary for a good information management system, people usually respond by discussing hardware and software. But equally critical to the success of any information system are the people or social context in which the system will operate. This dimension is sometimes referred to as "warmware." In clinical practice, perhaps more so than in highly automated facets of our society, warmware issues have been problematic.

Young physicians often complain that their formal medical training did not adequately prepare them for the realities of day-to-day practice. The diversity and complexity of patient care are reasons it is difficult to prepare fully for "real life" as a clinician. This same diversity and complexity, combined with the intense pressures and demands of medical practice, make it difficult to develop information products that fit smoothly into the flow of patient care. In the context of this complexity and the many dimensions of patient care, current electronic clinical information resources are less than optimal.

Why such resources are lacking is explained in part by considering how many different kinds of information-processing tasks are done in clinical practice, for example:

- Managing all the logistical aspects of running a practice
- Gathering and tracking many types of information about patients from many different sources
- Gathering medical knowledge from many different sources and combining this knowledge with patient data to make clinical decisions
- Implementing clinical decisions, which may include ordering tests, writing prescriptions, and educating patients.

We have a gut-level understanding about each of these processes and generally believe we do them pretty well. Such information processing, however, belongs to the realm of the "art" of medicine, which is highly complex and individual to the practitioner, and even the few intricate functions mentioned above are complexly intertwined. Unfortunately, no underlying "science" or even generally accepted conventions of clinical information processing can readily be used to evaluate and improve our information management activities. Similarly, the complexity, diversity, and individualized nature of clinical information management have been formidable obstacles for those attempting to develop practical and useful clinical information systems.

Nonetheless, much progress has been made during the last few decades in applying information technology to clinical practice. Understandably, these efforts have usually focused on relatively narrow and thus more manageable functions such as billing, prescription writing, digitizing popular textbooks, and the like. Robust knowledge bases are extremely difficult to develop and maintain owing to the vastness and rapid evolution of medical knowledge. Thus, available knowledge-based products generally have serious weaknesses, often in areas such as currency, comprehensiveness, or basis in evidence. Unfortunately, automating limited facets of a clinician's information world is problematic because there is so much interdependency between the various clinical information-processing functions. Even though some clinical computing applications have existed for decades, the fact that available products are not optimally integrated and not generally in widespread use (compared with magnetic resonance imaging, for example) suggests that, from the clinician's perspective, these tools are in an early stage of development.

You can make an analogy between the current state of clinical computing and personal banking before the introduction of automated teller machines (ATMs). Personal banking has been automated for some time, but the widespread use of ATM cards and devices made it markedly more convenient. Many factors should help accelerate the development of clinical information systems to a similar state of practicality. For example, standards and prototypes for computer-based records are being developed; many experts feel that automating patient data management is a prerequisite for ubiquitous clinical computing. Hardware and software are maturing rapidly, and computer tools are becoming more common in our daily, nonprofessional lives. In computer science generally and medicine specifically, expertise and

tools to make it easier to develop and maintain clinically useful knowledge bases are emerging.

Further stimulating this progress are external pressures mounting from payers, patients, and others for more evidence-based, patient-centered, outcome-driven care. Successfully meeting their demands will ultimately require the use of the technologies discussed in this book. At some point, each of these technologies or their offspring will play a crucial role in clinical information management. Today, many clinicians are using these products to great advantage in their daily practice. This book shows you why and how.

Making the Best of What Is Available

Evaluating Costs and Benefits

As with other decisions you make every day, successfully incorporating information technology into your practice requires a thoughtful assessment of the benefits and costs. A good place to begin is by reflecting on your current clinical information management practices. What types of information management tasks are most problematic for you, and what costs are you willing to bear to help solve these problems?

Just as patient management decisions are not based on consideration of a single option, the cost-benefit ratio for implementing various clinical information technologies must be considered in light of the alternatives. For example, deciding to build a medical CD-ROM library must be weighed against your current access to information resources (for example, textbooks and colleagues) and your propensity for asking and answering clinical questions.

Earlier, I noted several theoretical benefits of automating various clinical tasks—improving clinical efficiency and patient outcomes, increasing practice effectiveness and satisfaction, and others. While these advantages are difficult to evaluate or substantiate formally, they are reasonable guideposts to keep in mind as you contemplate implementing clinical information systems. The investments you must make to reap such benefits include the cost of procuring and maintaining the necessary hardware and software, the time spent learning to use the system, the time required to use the system at some point during your busy day, and the will to do things differently.

In the past, the energy required to yield a favorable return on a technologic investment has been considered so great that most physicians have simply not used the available information products. Currently, however, tools are rapidly evolving in the areas of utility and user-friendly interfaces. Costs are coming down. In addition, external pressures for state-of-the-art practices and outcomes are also growing rapidly. The changing dynamics of investment and return from using information technology suggest that the prudent course is to carefully and frequently reassess the use of computer-based products to support your clinical practice.

You can optimize the benefits of the information technology cost-benefit ratio if you focus first on an application area that is important but in some way deficient in your practice and for which good alternatives are lacking. For example, if literature searches are an important resource for your practice, but you find librarian-mediated searching not timely enough or not optimally effective, then pursuing literature searching on your own might be rewarding. Similarly, if most of the prescriptions you write come from a relatively small group of drugs, you might find that an integrated prescription management and patient drug information handout system would yield significant returns for the investment required. Once you have taken the initial plunge, adding other computer-based activities to your regular clinical computing repertoire should require less of an investment.

Now that telecommunication is becoming a part of everyday life (at least in the popular press if not in practice), you have a wonderful opportunity to hitch a ride onto the medical information superhighway. If you are contemplating the purchase of a home computer for general household purposes (for example, family entertainment, education, and so on), adding a modem and going online may then follow as a relatively painless way to begin exploring clinical computing applications. In fact, many households already use value-added telecommunication services such as CompuServe or Prodigy for financial and entertainment information, database resources, and many other kinds of offerings. Once you get online, medical telecommunications activities are just a short step away. You might consider looking into online resources for continuing medical education, literature searching, other medical databases for answering clinical questions, or online specialty forums such as ACP Online (the American College of Physicians' network for College members) for communicating with your colleagues. You can also easily begin exploring these types of products if your home unit is equipped with a CD-ROM drive. Even if your computer does not have a CD-ROM drive or a modem, you can still begin to sample useful medical software.

Selecting Useful Products

Each chapter in this guide seeks to familiarize you with the types of products available for a specific area of medical practice or information technology. Certain general strategies can be broadly useful as you approach the task of surveying the field, studying your options, and eventually implementing clinical information technology. These strategies include:

- Consulting computer-using colleagues
- Attending specialty meetings
- Looking into medical center resources
- Reading reviews and other supportive material
- Getting as much hands-on experience as possible.

To begin, look to your peers. Studies have shown that colleagues are a valuable resource for diffusing medical innovations and knowledge about them. Information technology is no exception. For example, a local colleague may have experience using a clinical information tool you are considering trying. In addition, online resources allow you to connect with others who are already experienced in areas you want to explore. Such colleagues can offer valuable tips on selecting and implementing products they are currently using. ACP Online has regular discussions about selecting and using portable computing devices and practice management software as well as other clinical computing topics. On a mailing list accessible via the Internet, one intrepid physician is regularly and extensively documenting his trials and tribulations in implementing a particular practice management software product.

National specialty meetings are also excellent for finding helpful colleagues who are successfully using information technology in their practices. In addition, many specialty society meetings offer courses on using clinical computing technology and give participants hands-on experience with various products. For example, ACP's Annual Session offers approximately 30 courses devoted to clinical uses of information technology, including a "Medical Informatics Resource Room" where participants can preview various clinical information technologies and discuss relevant issues with expert faculty. Vendors also show their wares in the traditional manner on the exhibit floor.

You might also want to look into the American Medical Informatics Association (AMIA), a membership organization dedicated to advancing the use of computers in health care. Extensive training, networking with colleagues, and hands-on opportunities are also available at AMIA's annual meeting each fall. Some specialty societies offer other services that help their members access and use clinical computing products. For example, ACP provides its members the opportunity to search the National Library of Medicine's MEDLINE and other databases for a flat yearly fee and offers discounts to members on selected clinical computing products from commercial vendors.

If you have access to an academic medical center

or residency training program, ask whether the medical school library or residency offices provide previewing of clinical software applications and contact with knowledgeable users. Recognizing that proficiency in using clinical information resources is becoming a critical skill for successful performance as a physician, the bodies that govern curricula for medical schools and residencies are encouraging greater attention to information management skills and products in the training process. Thus, most programs have ready access to at least literature-searching capabilities, and many offer access to other sophisticated information resources such as libraries on CD-ROM and diagnostic decision support programs.

Printed material, of course, should not be overlooked as a source for learning about clinical information technology. The book you are now reading should take you a long way in this direction. A companion book published by ACP and edited by Sue Frisch, *Software for Internists,* is a compendium of reviews of medical software that have previously appeared in *Medical Software Reviews (MSR)* as well as other medical journals. These reviews provide more information on the features of individual software products and their implementation. Ms. Frisch is the editor of *MSR,* an independent, monthly publication from Healthcare Computing Publications. Several other periodicals and catalogs also publish information related to the selection and clinical use of information technology.

Getting Started

The resources discussed in this book perform roughly four functions: 1) helping with the business management aspects of clinical practice; 2) supporting patient information flow in outpatient practice; 3) answering clinical questions; and 4) assisting with continued professional learning. Following are some general considerations for getting started with these different types of resources.

Business Management and Patient Information Flow

From the standpoint of implementation, business management and patient information flow functions have much in common. Systems that support either or both of these functions have a global effect on your practice. For example, installing practice management or medical record systems probably requires that several different computing devices be placed in different locations throughout your offices, and implementing these systems requires that essentially your entire staff be involved. These procedures will profoundly affect the logistics of your practice.

Similarly, implementing computer-based patient education, prescription management, and other systems that affect patient information flow may have broad implications for your practice. You must consider the effect of such systems on your practice and develop a plan to generate enthusiasm and obtain active support from your staff. Without support, your chances of reaping benefit from these systems is drastically diminished.

By contrast, implementing systems dedicated to clinical problem solving and educational growth is more a matter between you, the computer, and the software.

Answering Clinical Questions

Finding time to use information technology products during your overcrowded day will probably be a challenge. The better your new computer-based information products are incorporated into a natural work flow, the more likely you will be to use them. Over time, your work flow will evolve to include more efficient accessing of needed information.

A critical step in this integration is physically putting the computer and related devices in a convenient location. Think through the information-processing task you are trying to automate, and determine where the system will be most appropriately situated. Depending on the application and your practice, the best location might be your office; the examination, consultation, or lunch room; your home; or some other place. Many clinicians are successfully using computers in the presence of patients, but this issue must be carefully considered. Do not overlook ergonomic considerations such as adequate lighting and seating and proper placement of the keyboard, monitor, and other equipment. Remember that the goal is to lower the "activation energy barrier" to more easily integrate your new computer-based tools into everyday practice.

Your experience using computer-based tools for answering clinical questions will be more rewarding if you enhance the benefit component of the cost-benefit ratio. A landmark article (Covell DG, Uman GC, Manning PR. Information needs in office practice: are they being met? Ann Intern Med. 1985; 103:596-9) suggested that question-asking activity is directly related to the ease with which answers can be obtained. This same study illustrated that many information needs in office practice are unrecognized, and a majority are unanswered. Ready access to powerful clinical information resources such as those discussed throughout this book help to create a positive feedback loop, wherein successfully answering important clinical questions stimulates other important patient care questions to be asked and successfully answered.

For computer-based information resources to serve this function, however, several crucial steps must be negotiated. First, you must be able to recognize information needs as they occur and to frame a question based on those needs that can be posed to an information resource. Second, you must select an appropriate type of information resource, which may in fact *not* be computer-based. If a computer-based resource is appropriate, then you must choose the appropriate one. To do so, you must ask questions: Does the knowledge base of the product have the needed information? Is the knowledge base current, valid, evidence-based, and complete enough? Are the type and format of the information (for example, bibliographic citation versus free text versus lists of clinical findings or diseases) useful for solving the problem at hand? If your new computer-based information resource is the appropriate choice, you must then successfully use the program (that is, navigate the user interface, interpret the output, and so forth) to obtain the best that the resource has to offer.

Research with computer-based information tools has shown how problems can arise with each of the previously described steps. However, the better informed you are about the content and functionality of a particular information resource, the more likely you will be able to negotiate those information-access steps. A participant in a clinical computing study with which I was involved summarized the point succinctly: "System utility is directly proportional to training."

Many software users tend to pop open a software package, install it in the computer, and proceed directly to trying to use it, turning to the manual only when stumped. It has been argued that truly user-friendly systems should accommodate this type of "plug and play." I must caution against this method for most users of clinical computing products. Your investment in getting to know an information product well will be repaid with rewarding interactions and retrieval of useful information. Frustration and suboptimal information retrieval are the probable outcomes of not learning the system well.

Despite all the potential pitfalls, those familiar with computer-based information resources generally share the conviction that these products markedly improve the efficiency and effectiveness with which clinical questions are answered.

Continuing Medical Education

Using software successfully for continuing medical education (CME) involves many of the same issues as in answering clinical questions—the importance of training, the need for a current and complete knowledge base, and the potential for a "positive feedback loop." In fact, the process of answering clinical questions can be viewed as an important continuing education activity in its own right. Issues related to getting started with CME software are explored further in Chapter 7.

How To Use This Book

The Overall Plan

As described earlier, the purpose of this book is to help you make optimal use of available information technology products for supporting your management of clinical information. For the technologies discussed in the first ten chapters, we provide practical information for answering three specific questions:

- How can this technology help me in my practice?
- What types of commercial products are currently available?
- How can I successfully implement this technology in my practice?

Accordingly, each of the first ten chapters is divided into three sections. An eleventh chapter covers some of the fundamentals of hardware and software. Computer novices may wish to begin with the last chapter, the terms and concepts of which are used in most chapters of the book. The glossary contains definitions for common and some not-so-common terms relevant to general and clinical computing; it is, however, limited to the terms used in this book. Finally, the Appendix provides pointers to additional helpful resources such as organizations, publications, and software.

Contents of the Chapters

The available medical information technology products are divided into ten categories, discussed individually in Chapters 1 through 10.

1. PRACTICE MANAGEMENT deals with technology designed to automate the business aspects of an outpatient medical practice. The third section of this chapter provides a step-by-step implementation strategy that can also be applied to medical record systems and other office-wide automation activities.

2. MEDICAL RECORD SYSTEMS FOR OFFICE PRACTICE, closely related to Chapter 1, focuses on technology that can be used to automate the processing of a wide range of patient information in the outpatient setting.

3. MEDICAL LITERATURE MANAGEMENT presents the fundamentals of electronically accessing and searching the medical literature using your personal computer. The chapter then readdresses the three questions in terms of available literature-filing products, namely, the bibliographic database managers.

4. DIAGNOSTIC DECISION SUPPORT discusses in detail four commercial programs that illustrate the utility and use of this category of software. The theoretical and practical aspects of these diagnostic programs are compared. (Readers unfamiliar with this technology may wish to focus initially on the first and third sections of the chapter for an overview.)

5. THERAPEUTIC DECISION SUPPORT covers a broad range of software that can be used to help the clinician develop and implement patient management strategies. Therapeutic functions discussed in this chapter include selecting therapies, obtaining drug information, writing and tracking prescriptions, checking drug interactions, and prescribing and evaluating diet therapy.

6. PATIENT EDUCATION reviews the ingredients of successful patient education strategies and provides information on using software to support these activities.

7. PERSONAL CONTINUING MEDICAL EDUCATION discusses how available software products can help make your CME activities more convenient and cost-effective.

8. TELECOMMUNICATIONS addresses the functionality available within online systems and the ways you can use these systems to support your clinical communication and information-gathering activities.

9. CD-ROM TECHNOLOGY AND FULL-TEXT INFORMATION RETRIEVAL helps you understand the hardware and software products necessary to build and use your own clinical libraries on disk.

10. PORTABLE COMPUTING DEVICES provides an overview of the use and utility of small devices ranging from palmtop computers to personal digital assistants (PDAs) and subnotebook computers.

The final chapter, COMPUTER BASICS, introduces the reader to basic yet practical issues in understanding, buying, and using computer-related products.

Caveats for the Reader

Creating categories of commercial clinical computing products and answering the three questions for each category are not straightforward tasks. Several complexities arising from these activities are described below, and understanding them will help you make the best use of this book.

Categorizing the Products

First, many available information-processing functions do not fit into neat, mutually exclusive categories.

Thus, information relevant to an important topic may appear in several places throughout this book. For example, literature searching is discussed in detail in Chapter 3, but the main routes for performing this function (that is, with online systems and CD-ROM) are discussed in detail in Chapters 8 and 9. Similarly, patient education handouts are discussed in detail in Chapter 6, but since practice management, medical record, and therapeutic decision support systems may also generate such handouts, they are also mentioned in Chapters 1, 2, and 5.

Furthermore, while the technology discussed in a particular chapter may consist primarily of software (for example, therapeutic decision support) or hardware (for example, portable computing devices), a variable mixture of hardware and software issues are discussed in each chapter. Despite these interrelationships, we have attempted to make each chapter stand on its own. Rich cross-referencing and indexing, however, have been developed to assist you in gathering all the information you may need on a particular topic.

Answering the Three Questions

The three questions posed in each of the first ten chapters—how can this technology help me, what types of products are available, and how can I implement them—have proved surprisingly difficult to answer definitively. Several factors combine to make difficult the successful description of clinical computing resources. Included among these factors are the relatively limited diffusion of each technology into routine clinical practice, the large number of different products that have been competing for this

limited use, the great speed of hardware and software evolution, and the relatively limited publicity for successful clinical implementations.

The model we used to create this book, namely, answering the three questions based on the authors' experiences and research, may limit somewhat the breadth of the material provided. To broaden the perspective, however, the editor used several online bulletin boards and mailing lists that reach many hundreds of computer-knowledgeable clinicians to invite other physicians to comment on the answers to these questions. In an additional effort to broaden the input, the editor sent each of the chapters to two different peer reviewers for constructive feedback. The thoughtful feedback from the few who responded to the online queries and from each of the reviewers was helpful in refining the presentation of material. However, it is interesting to note that relatively little additional content was provided by these supplementary sources.

Providing Product-Specific Information

Since this book is intended to offer a practical overview of the utility and use of available *types* of clinical information management resources, we have not attempted to provide a comprehensive or up-to-the-minute catalog of available clinical information products. In fact, so rapid is the evolution of medical information technology that it is likely that many (if not most) of the products discussed will be available in an updated and perhaps significantly modified version by the time you read this guide.

It is also important to note that the products discussed in each chapter have been selected by the chapter author(s) to illustrate the different functionality currently available in commercial information products. Authors primarily used their working knowledge of available products to provide these illustrations; they were not asked to formally survey, evaluate, and update their knowledge of all products in a given category before writing their chapter.

Similarly, the Appendix provides the interested reader with additional information for pursuing the topics discussed in the book. The sampling of organizations, publications, services, products, and the like will convey a sense of the current state of the art in clinical computing trends and technologies. We believe that clinicians will find among these resources some that prove useful in planning, purchasing, and implementing a computer-based clinical information management system.

Finally, ACP has neither formally reviewed any of the products mentioned in this book nor attempted to make sure that all products available in each category are mentioned. Thus, inclusion or exclusion of any specific product should not be construed as a reflection by ACP or the editor on the value of the product for clinical use. We hope that the material presented by the authors convinces you that the technologies discussed can be useful and that you can successfully implement them. The product-specific information presented throughout this guide is intended to stimulate your further inquiry into the state of the art and the status of individual products at the time of your reading. The techniques mentioned earlier in this introduction to identify and evaluate available programs should assist you in this task.

These considerations notwithstanding, we believe that *Computers in Clinical Practice* is the most complete single resource available for understanding the clinical relevance of information technology and providing answers to the key implementation questions. We trust that this book will become a valuable resource for clinicians and others interested in better managing the explosive growth and complexity of clinical information. ACP is currently exploring strategies for delivering regularly updated versions of this material to physicians as well as for delivering more current and comprehensive information about specific commercial products. These efforts are part of ACP's ongoing and growing commitment to offer products and services that help practitioners understand and use clinical information technology.

1

PRACTICE MANAGEMENT

Matthew Cushing, MD, FACP

HOW CAN PRACTICE MANAGEMENT SYSTEMS HELP ME IN MY PRACTICE?

Computers are widely used in our society to improve the management efficiency of businesses. However, many physicians are not yet benefiting from the varied ways in which computerized office management can increase efficiency and improve health care delivery in everyday practice. This chapter looks at some of the advantages to computerizing practice management, presents some specific programs dedicated to this end, and discusses the implementation of these systems in practical terms.

CLAIMS TRACING. How often have you sent an insurance claim to the carrier, only to have it seem-ingly vanish? You have no idea where it is or whether the carrier received it. In addition, weeks or months might elapse before you become aware of its loss—unless you are reminded. With an office computer system, however, the reminders are automatic, and you can electronically query the third party and receive an immediate reply. Further, you can electronically check your claim for "red flags" such as incompatible procedure or diagnosis code pairs before you submit it.

PATIENT INFORMATION. How many of your female patients over 25 years of age have not had a Papanicolaou smear in 2 years? Which patients with diabetes are behind on their glucose level tests and fundus checks? Who needs a diphtheria-tetanus booster? Which patient with a positive purefied protein derivative (PPD) test for tuberculosis was lost to follow-up? What about following up on the patient

1

with the borderline mammogram result? Unless you can flexibly and readily access your patient data, you may miss timely answers to these and many other crucial questions, putting both your patients and yourself at risk. With computerization, follow-up on patient information becomes more automatic.

RISK MANAGEMENT. Every risk management consultant will tell you that the best defense against liability is meticulous record keeping. Document everything. Unfortunately, detailed record keeping can be tedious without a computer. With a computerized system, however, you do not have to document in free text that you advised the patient on the risks and benefits for each test or treatment ordered, or that the patient was alert and appeared to comprehend and that you provided the advice to the patient in writing. Risk management record keeping becomes an easier and less time-consuming task.

ELECTRONIC BILLING. Management consultants will tell you that replacing a person with a machine saves money. Machines do not take vacations, require health insurance, retire, or have moods. Insurance companies, too, have discovered this fact. They would much rather obtain data electronically than pay a keypunch operator to enter it. In addition, the error rate is markedly reduced when you transmit your billing data by telephone, and the insurance companies then reward you with less hassle, faster turnaround time, and, therefore, quicker payments.

DATA STORAGE AND RETRIEVAL. Electronic data storage has many advantages over paper systems. You can index, search, reorganize, and retrieve the data more quickly and easily. Under adequate pass-word protection, electronic data storage is much more secure than paper records. You can archive and store all data off the premises, making them impervious to fire, flood, and earthquake damage. Storage of data can be accomplished in a tiny fraction of the space required for paper. One optical disk (which is similar to a CD-ROM [compact disc–read-only memory]) can hold the equivalent of shelf after shelf of patient records. Further, all printed materials you receive in the mail or by fax can be scanned into the electronic storage medium.

MANAGED CARE REQUIREMENTS. Managed care is now entering the outpatient medical arena, causing questions to be raised about proper documentation, preventive medicine, patient information, and so forth. Managed care requirements make a paper record system awkward and labor intensive. Not only are electronic data easier to find than data in paper systems, but reminders can also be programmed into your computer system to ensure that each patient is asked to keep up with proper scheduling for preventive care and is reminded when she or he forgets. In addition, as prepayment becomes more popular, you will need to figure your costs and revenues on a per-patient-encounter basis, a job made much easier with a computer.

MEDICAL EQUIPMENT PURCHASE DECISIONS AND PRACTICE MARKETING. Spreadsheets let you play with alternatives for each decision involving cost-benefit concerns. You enter the costs and fees in your program, and then see what volume you need to break even or enter the black with each procedure or service before you commit any funds or personnel to it. For example, if you are considering a purchase of testing equipment, you could then create a model on your spreadsheet as follows: You show income based on allowable fees, multiplied by a variable called "number of tests per period," and show expenses (the total of capitalization, interest on loans, supplies, repairs, salaries, and fringe benefits of lab personnel), multiplied by the number of hours per week required to operate the equipment. Next you estimate the time required to set up and clean the equipment, run standards and controls, and keep a log. Then you alter the variable number-of-tests factor to see how many tests you would need to do in a given period to break even. This technique gives you an idea of whether the equipment would be self-supporting. Besides cost-benefit analyses, you can also use your computer system to remind patients of the services you offer and to target patient groups by demographics to receive flyers, bulletins, and informational handouts.

TIME MANAGEMENT. You can use computer programs to cross-schedule resources. For example, you can schedule flexible sigmoidoscopy or Holter monitoring so that it is available at a time when the personnel are free to operate it and so that more than one patient is not scheduled to use the same equipment at the same time. Furthermore, you can use the computer to keep your personal schedule and to beep you to remind you of appointments. The computer can generate a to-do list and schedule projects flexibly, and it can even create a "Gantt chart," showing overlapping timelines for each section of a large project, for example, building a new office.

WHAT COMPUTERIZED PRACTICE MANAGEMENT PRODUCTS ARE AVAILABLE?

Although more than 400 systems are being sold in today's market, most have little to recommend them. I have reviewed a few dozen systems, enough to have an overview of what the market is like. I think that many systems were designed either by amateur programmers, who really do not have the skills to write sophisticated programs, or by good programmers who have no idea of the problems physicians meet in running a practice. Remember that writing a good medical system program is a complicated undertaking, requiring thousands of man-hours. That is why there are few, if any, good, comprehensive systems that are also inexpensive.

What Makes a Good System?

First, a good system is based on the programmer's knowledge of how a medical office works and his or her willingness to make the system fit in with the office routine, not disrupt it. A quick, reliable interface with the users and fast, intuitive data-entry capabilities are essential. Most office management programs have not yet adopted graphical user interfaces (GUIs), which are becoming standard with consumer software. A program should employ accepted standards of computer keyboard usage rather than a new and obscure system of keystrokes to operate the software. Data should be visible at a glance and easily changeable (where it is safe to be so). Reports should be easy to design and should contain the data you want to see. Your practice management system should be able to generate a complex report in a few minutes, not hours. Flexibility is critical. The data you store and the format you use should be adaptable to your practice style and type. Finally, internal checking should be a part of the program to prevent arithmetical errors.

Get recommendations from colleagues, but be mindful of who says what. While user endorsement is valuable, it is far from foolproof. Doctors tend to be paternalistic about their own systems. After all, when you have spent thousands of dollars on office management software and hardware, admitting to a mistake in choice is difficult. However, office person-

nel, who do not have a financial or emotional stake in the investment, tend to be more honest about the drawbacks, and, as a rule, they use the system more than the physician does. Consult those who know.

From among the plethora of available systems, I have selected a handful of known, good programs for mention. A list of these programs is given in Table 1-1. The Appendix provides references to product reviews, which offer a more detailed analysis of individual practice management systems, as well as to other useful resources.

All of the products noted below are rated at least fair in the areas of data entry, report generation, flexibility, and error checking. Some, however, excel in individual areas. For example, Medical Manager has excellent error-checking capability and The Resident is highly flexible.

Table 1-1. Practice Management Products Discussed

Product	Platform	Manufacturer	Publisher or Address	Phone and Fax Numbers
MDX	UNIX, AIX	Physician Computer Network, Inc./Calyx	16745 Bluemound Road Suite 200 Brookfield, WI 53008	Tel: 414-782-0300 Fax: 414-782-3182
Medical Manager	DOS, UNIX, AIX, XENIX	Systems Plus, Inc.	500 Clyde Avenue Mountain View, CA 94043	Tel: 415-969-7047 Fax: 415-969-0118
PAL/MED	DOS, UNIX, AIX, XENIX, Windows	Medical Synergies Corp.	4360 Chamblee Dunwoody Road Suite 400 Atlanta, GA 30341	Tel: 800-285-8602 Fax: 404-458-0319
Practice Partner, Medical Billing	DOS, UNIX	Physician Micro Systems, Inc.	2033 Sixth Avenue Suite 707 Seattle, WA 98121	Tel: 206-441-8490 Fax: 206-441-8915
The Resident	UNIX	Physician Computer Network, Inc.	1200 The American Road Morris Plains, NJ 07950	Tel: 201-490-3100 Fax: 201-490-3101

Medical Manager

Medical Manager (Figure 1-1) is a venerable program, one of the earliest on the market, and is now in its eighth version. It offers a very good office management system and a fairly good clinical record system. The program suffers from lack of a seamless word processing connection, and the report generator is fussy and hard to use, but Medical Manager is the number-one seller among programs of its type in the United States.

The Resident

This system from Physician Computer Network, Inc., combines an excellent and versatile office management system with a new clinical data system. The older clinical data module was fairly limited, but the new release may be much better. This system is worth considering but may not be easy to find because vendors are scattered.

MDX

This office management system is adequate; the user interface is not the best, but it does the job. Physician Computer Network, Inc., a New Jersey–based corporation, has acquired the publisher. You should clarify this point if you contact them.

Practice Partner

Practice Partner is a good all-purpose system. It has a built-in word processor, but the text formatting is based on older "dot codes," which must be embedded in the text; it also lacks many of the sophisticated features of the latest commercial word processors. Versyss Corporation, a marketer of medical office management software, claims an affiliation by which they are going to use the clinical data

```
04/14/93          Personalized Programming, Inc.          Menu 1
                        The Medical Manager
                  Sydney Carrington & Associates 8.01

  1 - NEW Patient Entry          7 - FILE Maintenance

  2 - PROCEDURE Entry            8 - OFFICE Management

  3 - PAYMENT Entry              9 - SYSTEM Utilities

  4 - DISPLAY Patient Data      10 - CUSTOM Menus

  5 - REPORT Generation         11 - MANAGED Care

  6 - BILLING & EDI             12 - ADVANCED Systems

              Enter Desired Option: .....
```

```
04/14/93            Managed Care System            CMenu 33
                 Sydney Carrington & Associates 8.01

  1 - Referral To Specialist       7 - Define Plan Contract

  2 - Referral To Facility         8 - Maintain Eligibility Roster

  3 - Referrals Received           9 - Managed Care Utilities

  4 - Post Capitation Payments    10 - (Reserved)

  5 - Edit Capitation Payments    11 - Managed Care Reports

  6 - (Reserved)                  12 - Managed Care Parameters

              Enter Desired Option: .....
```

Figure 1-1. Medical Manager. Top. A menu of different program options. **Bottom.** A menu of managed care system options.

module of Practice Partner in combination with Versyss' office management system, Mends, and WordPerfect to create a complete clinical and business system. This combination will be worth a look.

PAL/MED

A new version of this product is expected after this writing. If it contains all of the features its developer promises, it could be excellent and certainly worth serious consideration. PAL/MED is a complete office management system, seamlessly combining clinical data with billing.

HOW CAN I SUCCESSFULLY IMPLEMENT PRACTICE MANAGEMENT SYSTEMS IN MY OFFICE?

Should you start using a computerized practice management system in your office now? Not surprisingly, many factors must be considered before making such an important decision.

Reasons for Starting Now

Waiting for New Technology Is Pointless

Technology is always improving. No matter when you buy a system, if you wait a few more months, you can buy one with more features that is easier to use and probably cheaper.

So why should you buy a system now? Becoming familiar with any system takes time, and the benefits of computerization depend on your using its capabilities as soon as possible. Time is not on your side. The longer you wait, the longer it takes for you to establish the skills and information needed to cope with the challenges of the 1990s and beyond.

Managed Care Makes Computerization Essential

In the future, I think it is possible that physicians will be penalized economically as well as in reputation unless they run a very smart business, one with all of the features and hallmarks of sophisticated medical practice. These features will include:

- Every patient being appropriately educated about the benefits of preventive medicine

- Automatic ticklers on periodic tests and follow-ups

- Instant statistics on patients needing reminders and quickly generated reminder letters

- Electronic exchange of information with managed care organizations and other payers.

I predict that within a decade most "reimbursement" will be prepaid, per patient per month, with a base figure and multipliers. The multipliers will depend in part on how many objective criteria of excellence your practice can generate, based on quality-control standards. You had better be ready. You can possibly comply without computers in a small practice with a large staff, but if you can only afford fewer than four or five staff members per physician, you should consider computerization of your data.

Becoming Familiar with Computerized Systems Is Important

As I have already mentioned, the learning curve is steep at first. You must feel that you are in charge of your system, that you can master it and feel comfortable with all of its features. If you feel intimidated, the system will take control rather than you controlling it. Thus, the sooner you get started, the better.

Hardware Is Cheap and Reliable

Hardware systems may get cheaper, but their performance/price ratios are excellent. Hard disks have superior reliability, as do memory chips. In addition, backing up your data regularly provides excellent insurance against the unlikely event of hardware failure. If you are a novice in regard to computers, read about the fundamentals of hardware in Chapter 11 of this book.

Difficulties and Misgivings in Getting Started

Vendors May Be Unreliable

SOME VENDORS ARE UNSCRUPULOUS. Vendors want to make a profit. Potential clients who are not familiar with computer technology can be easily bamboozled with technobabble and a glib demonstration. This type of presentation can hide serious defects in the knowledge and training of the vendor's staff. Even more important, many vendors make a practice of stalling when a user calls with a problem that is hard to solve or appears at an inconvenient time. In addition, pricing may bear little or no relationship to the vendor's costs and may be based more on the "deep pockets" theory, especially regarding maintenance and upgrade costs.

MANY VENDORS ARE INCOMPETENT. Although vendors have to know something about the systems they sell to install them and to get you to buy, their knowledge of the roots of the system (operating system and hardware) may be sketchy. The installation process, if sloppily done, can leave your hard disk cluttered with many useless, temporary installation files and files that are never used again. Furthermore, cables are frequently left unlabeled and sometimes not grounded, creating potential hazards for the future.

MANY VENDORS ARE SHORT-HANDED. Training employees is expensive for the vendor, and pay in the industry tends to be low, with limited advancement. Consequently, employee turnover is high. An owner might choose to leave a vacant position unfilled rather than train a new employee on a complex system. Therefore, when you call for help or training, you may be ignored or stalled.

Operating Systems Still Have Problems

Even the most popular operating systems may be rather unfriendly and problematic for some users. UNIX sometimes shuts down mysteriously, with no clear explanation of what has gone wrong. Networks are subject to quirky intermachine communication and frustrating delays. Commands are often written by programmers for programmers and are far from intuitive (for example, UNIX commands like "cat," "grep," and "ps" are hardly self-explanatory). Error messages can be all but indecipherable and very intimidating (for example, "Memory fault. Core dumped" or "Error 105 at CB45:1077").

Hardware Problems Still Exist

Notwithstanding a high level of excellence in the computer hardware industry, all is not perfect. Printer interfaces are not standardized, and a printer can simply quit, sometimes with little overt indication of what is wrong. Cables work loose, and the equipment stops. Static electricity can corrupt your data; back-up tape drives become balky or slow; data on floppy disks are subject to many hazards. If you do not have the time and patience to deal with such problems, you may begin to feel overwhelmed.

Self-Installation Has Pitfalls

The main problem with a do-it-yourself computer system is that you are using valuable time for work that someone else can do better—time that you could use to greater advantage in your professional life. And problems in these systems can demand incredible amounts of time (for example, trying to configure a serial printer, re-indexing a corrupted data file, figuring out the proper terminal emulator to use, or tracking down an errant TTY file). If you cannot figure out whether a balky system is in trouble because of hardware or software, and you bought them from different sources, you can be sure that the hardware dealer will blame the problem on the software and vice versa.

Step-by-Step Implementation

Although getting started can be difficult, your initial success depends almost entirely on two factors: picking the right vendor of good software and knowing enough about the requirements of a good system to be able to oversee installation and training knowledgeably. As must be clear by now, a good dealer can be a valuable asset.

With common sense, adaptability, and the intelligence that enabled you to survive 20 years of training and competition, you can accomplish this project in a manner that will enhance not only the efficiency, but also the pleasure, of your practice for many years. A recommended nine-step approach to the implementation of a new system is given in the following sections. The nine steps are:

1. Preparing a list of requirements
2. Deciding on a purchase plan
3. Picking likely software candidates
4. Choosing a dealer
5. Evaluating systems
6. Selecting a system
7. Purchasing your system
8. Agreeing to terms: the contract
9. Installing and using your system.

Step 1. Preparing a List of Requirements

This step, so often omitted, is critical. Do not neglect the 30 minutes it takes to think through the following items; then make a simple one-page summary to share with the dealer.

NUMBER OF PRACTICE SITES. Are you planning to run more than one office site? If so, you should plan telephone communications between your sites and will have to dedicate at least one line to this purpose.

If you are using a network as your operating system, you may need more than one line.

NUMBER OF PHYSICIANS. The number of physicians you plan to employ determines the size of your practice, the amount of clinical data you want to store, and the number of independent data-entry and retrieval sites you need. Also, each physician should probably have at least one printer.

NUMBER AND KINDS OF EMPLOYEES. Think ahead a couple of years. How many receptionists and book-keepers will you need? How many office nurses? You need to know this information to provide for the number of users on the system and to run cables to most potential work sites.

BILLING METHODS. Are you planning to do your own billing? Will you bet on fee-for-service being the preferred method of reimbursement in your practice for the next few years? Will you send your bills electronically (initial higher cost but much faster and more reliable returns)? Will you be doing patient billing, or will most bills be sent to third parties?

PRESCRIPTION REQUIREMENTS. Do you have many patients on long-term therapy? If so, you are probably caught in the trap of having to write two to three copies each of several prescriptions—for example, one to send away, a local one in the meantime, and one to take on vacation. Moreover, keeping track of prescription refills, quantity, duration, and so forth is time consuming, especially if the request comes when you are out of the office. Your program should keep track of this information for you and also flag drug interactions and allergies with minimal effort. A practice management system with an appropriate clinical module can handle all of those chores effort-lessly. Your requirements in this area (and several mentioned below) will give you a sense of whether you should be looking for a medical record system (see Chapter 2) in addition to a practice management system.

RECORD STORAGE METHODS. Will you store hand-written or typed notes in the traditional way, or do you want to have computer access to transcriptions of dictated notes? The latter gives you much quicker access and saves the labor of constantly procuring and refiling charts, but you will need far larger computer storage capacity for free text. If you want to use a scanner to enter outside data such as imaging and cardiology reports into the computer, then plan on an even larger capacity. Allow at least 500 megabytes (Mb) for each doctor employed in your practice if you plan to use computer-stored patient records. Storing your patient records on optical discs (similar to CD-ROMs) is now possible and is economical to do once the system to record the discs is in place.

TYPE OF NOTES. The amount of space you need to store clinical records is directly proportional to the amount of free text you plan to create. Several hundred Mb per user is mandatory for average-length clinical text. The space requirement depends on which of three options you choose: dictated free text primarily, some dictated text with checklists, or checklists with handwritten notes.

LABORATORY INPUT TO OFFICE. Will you be doing your tests in an office lab? If so, you may want to consider direct input of data into your medical record system. This requires special connections—an RS488 bus (HPIB, GPIB) as a rule—to your system.

REFERENCE LABORATORIES. Larger reference laboratories are willing, in exchange for a large volume of business, to send data by telephone line, either to a dedicated printer in your office or, even better, directly into your computer system to give you instant access to results. Labs that have already shown a willingness to do this are SmithKline, Metpath/Damon, Abbott, and Bioran. Get in touch with your reference laboratory if this feature is important to you.

REPORT INPUT. If you plan to have computer access to outside reports, you will need a scanner to feed the images into your electronic record and software to store and retrieve the images. Items you might consider saving include imaging reports (for example, from x-rays, ultrasounds, computed tomographic images, and magnetic resonance images), consultation letters, and hospital inpatient records, among others.

PRINTER REQUIREMENTS. The absolute minimum printer requirement is a fast dot-matrix machine for reports and bills, but you will probably want a laser or ink-jet printer for polished-looking copy.

Step 2. Deciding on a Purchase Plan

RESELLER OR DIRECT PURCHASE? The basic question to ask yourself is whether you are going to buy off-the-shelf hardware and software and install them yourself or whether you want to guard against the problems of self-installation by buying through a reseller (dealer) and having him or her do the installation. Some publishers accept the do-it-yourself option and will give you instructions for loading their software. Most discourage the practice. Although buying off the shelf saves you the dealer mark-up on your purchase, you can be left without resources when (not if) something goes wrong. Do not consider the latter option unless you love tinkering with computers and feel at home troubleshooting computer systems.

Step 3. Picking Likely Software Candidates

CHECK YOUR RESOURCES. Earlier in this chapter, I listed a few names of programs with which to get started. (You can also consult the information resources in the Appendix of this book.) Another good source of program names is your local computer-using colleagues, especially local internists. All you need to know from other users at this stage is whether they like the software they use and the name and telephone number of the publisher or a distributor. Unless you find a likely candidate from these resources, start with the systems I mentioned above (*see under* What Computerized Practice Management Products Are Available?).

CALL PUBLISHERS; GET LOCAL DEALERS. Publishers' lists of dealers are often out of date or simply wrong. Dealers go out of business or drop product lines or the marketing department has incorrect telephone numbers. In any case, you need to get as many dealer names and telephone numbers within an hour's drive of your office as you can.

GET PRICES FOR SOFTWARE FROM THE PUBLISHER. Publishers can and will stonewall on prices: They may say that "it depends on dealer markup" and the like. But you should insist on a ballpark figure or, better, the price charged to the dealer. After all, the publisher is (or should be) interested in making a sale. Frankly, if you assert that this information is essential to your making an informed decision, most publishers will be forthright about their price. You should also get information on total sales to date. The programs I have mentioned all have substantial sales, but they do vary (from Medical Manager, the nation's bestseller, to some with only a few hundred installations).

Step 4. Choosing a Dealer

Call Local Dealers

Once you get and confirm telephone numbers for local dealers, you can begin the winnowing process. Unless at least two or three dealers in your area can confirm that they carry the software and will install it, you had better broaden your horizons and look elsewhere. I feel strongly about this because of my previous experience with dealers. In spite of all your preparation and inquiries, you may find that after some time your dealer fails to satisfy you in some manner. Unless you have a choice of dealers, you would have to convert or re-enter data into another system, which would be a major inconvenience—if not a disaster. If one or two other dealers are in the area, you can also use the threat of switching to help settle your differences with your current dealer. At worst, you will have a back-up dealer to contact.

Get the Names of Three Nearby Users from the Dealer

Resist the pressure for a visit and demonstration from the salesman at this point, but do insist on getting the names and office telephone numbers of three internist or family practice users nearby who have been with the dealer for at least a year. Tell the dealer that without such a list no purchases will be made. Call each user on the list and speak to the office manager or bookkeeper. Ask if you and your office manager could visit for about an hour. If the answer is yes, make an appointment. Talk to the most knowledgeable office employee—the one who uses the program most often and is familiar with all of its functions, for example, registration, scheduling, billing and posting, and report generation.

Rate the Program and the Dealer

During your visit with the knowledgeable user, ask a lot of questions. Specifically, request a rating of the program and the dealer on the following areas.

USER INTERFACE. How easy is it to see data at a glance? Can a patient's data be called up quickly and easily? Can data be edited rapidly? Can you move from one part of the program to another seamlessly and within a second or two? Is the screen easy to peruse at a glance?

VERSATILITY AND CUSTOMIZATION. When third-party requirements change, can the data be altered to fit their format, both on paper and electronically? Can all codes be changed easily (codes for procedures, diagnoses, place and type of service, insurance identifiers, and so forth)? Can the program handle both fee-for-service and prepayment (capitation) in any combination? Does it allow you to post to several claims centers for the same carrier? Can you adjust fee schedules easily for Gramm-Rudman factors, deductibles, coinsurance, and the like? Can you design your own forms and reports?

THIRD-PARTY AND PATIENT BILLING. Can the office generate paper and electronic bills easily, and do the third-party bills contain every detail of information necessary to make clear what you did and why? For patient bills, are all the data in easily understood statements? Do patient bills show who owes what and why? Is there room to add a statement to patient bills and modifiers and explanations to insurance bills?

REPORT GENERATION. Are the users able to generate reports on all aspects of their patient's financial data, including managed care items like referrals, hospitalizations, and outside tests? Can they customize reports, such as requesting sorting by carrier, by date billed, and by date last posted to? Does the program show charges and receipts by procedure, by doctor, by facility, by diagnosis? Can they see at a glance the allowable charge by procedure for each carrier? Can their aging accounts summary list by date of procedure and by date of posting? Can they design a quick custom report with accurate results?

DATA SECURITY AND CONFIDENTIALITY. What provisions are incorporated into the software to ensure that your practice data remain secure and confidential? Is there an audit trail for changes made to critical data? Are passwords required for access to clinical or otherwise confidential information? Does the system ensure that "good" passwords are chosen (for example, passwords of more than three characters, including letters and other types of characters)? Are users "logged out" of a terminal when it is idle, even if only for a few moments?

SERVICE AND SUPPLIES. Does the vendor supply promptly and at a reasonable cost all computer peripherals and supplies as needed?

RESPONSIVENESS TO PROBLEMS. How fast and effective is the dealer in response to reported problems? Can the users get help for a problem any time the office is open, including 4:30 p.m. on the Friday before a holiday weekend? Do they get a quick callback on problems? Can the dealer handle most problems and almost all software problems by telephone access to his or her computer?

VALUE FOR COST OF PROGRAM AND SUPPORT SERVICES. Do they feel that their system saves them enough money and time to justify the outlay?

Step 5. Evaluating Systems

INVOLVE YOUR STAFF! One of the commonest errors in purchasing a computer system is to act on one's own and buy a system "for the good of the staff." First, they will feel patronized. Second, they will consider it "your" system instead of "our" system, and then, when a problem occurs, instead of helping to fix it, they will complain and feel alienated. At any rate, your staff will use the system far more often than you will, so they should have a say in selection and implementation.

GET ALL DEALER STATEMENTS ON PAPER. Whenever the dealer makes an initial presentation, preferably without a demonstration, take notes. Write down as much as you can of the dealer's statements and assertions and have your notes typed. Then send them to the dealer with a request to review and sign them if he or she agrees that it is an accurate reflection of the statements made, or have the dealer change any statements that he or she cannot support and then sign. These assertions should also be incorporated into the contract (*see under* Step 8), thus avoiding many misunderstandings and overstatements.

BE SURE TO COVER EVERY ITEM ON THE PERSONAL LIST YOU CREATED IN STEP 1. The configuration of your system depends on the decisions you made about the items on your personal list of requirements—the location and kind of hardware, the size of storage capacity, the number of modems and ports required, and much more. Be sure that the dealer handles each of these items.

SERVICE AND SUPPLIES. Spell out what you expect the dealer to do and provide. Do you want to buy your own supplies and probably save money, or do you want to get the dealer to provide them for your convenience? Frankly, dealers have little interest in this—their profit is low, and they have to keep inventory. But it is worth considering.

SERVICE AGREEMENTS. These are crucial to good performance. The agreement should state in detail that the dealer is responsible for making the system work as advertised and that for a monthly fee she or he will continue to do so, *whether the problem resides in hardware or in software, including the operating system and peripherals (modems, cables, and so on).* Furthermore, you should delineate what constitutes proper response time, including at night, on weekends, and on holidays; and you should insist on monetary or other tangible rewards and penalties based on adherence to these agreements. Anything less will result in frustration and anger and could be disastrous.

SOFTWARE UPGRADES. Most software publishers come out with approximately annual upgrades. Your maintenance contract should specify free upgrades to the software as each version comes out. All major publishers continually improve their product based on user feedback and availability of new software capabilities; you should be afforded the results whenever they become available. In all fairness, it should be said that upgrades have a down side: They are almost invariably infected with software "bugs." In my system, for example, the list of bugs in the most recent upgrade ran to two pages of single-spaced text. Discuss this factor with your dealer before signing up for the upgrades, and be sure you understand the procedure for addressing bugs in new program versions before making your decision.

COST AND AVAILABILITY OF SUPPLIES. Spell out in the maintenance agreement exactly what supplies are covered and check in a standard computer supply catalog to be sure that you are not paying more than about 120% of the catalog prices. Also, ask the dealer how much inventory he is planning to keep and whether other clients have a similar agreement.

WARRANTY. I think that a warranty without penalties is fairly useless. I suggest you try to set up a sliding scale for the maintenance agreement costs based on a standard of performance—fast and accurate gets maximum reimbursement.

Never settle for less than a 6-month warranty on the whole system, and at least a 1-year warranty on hardware, especially the printer, keyboard, mouse, cables, and modem. The warranty should allow you an option to back out if, for example, after a month's trial you find that the system does not suit you. Expect to have to pay for the dealer's time for installation and training. That is only fair. The warranty should stipulate that the system should operate as advertised and as stated in the presentation and demonstration; that errors and operating delays should be corrected within, at most, 2 business days (1 day would be better); and that any delay beyond that should be compensated by a monetary penalty. After all, your time is worth money, too. Do not let the dealer foist the hardware warranty onto the manufacturer. This is often done. The contract should state that it is the dealer's responsibility to negotiate with manufacturers and to provide you with a back-up unit in case of problems.

Step 6. Selecting a System

QUANTITATE OR GRAPH USER COMMENTS. Be sure that you numerically rate users' answers to the above questions (*see under* Step 4). Then display the results visually in a table or chart so that you can see at a glance the strong and weak points of each installation. You might assign higher point ranges to areas of particular concern to you (for example, promptness). Drawing bar graphs is often helpful to show the strong and weak points of each system in each office. (If you have a spreadsheet, this task can be automated with a few keystrokes.)

USE ONE DEALER TO RATE ANOTHER'S PRODUCT. Dealers may be overly optimistic about their own products, but they are usually on target when detailing the weaknesses of the competition. Of course, you should verify the negative comments, but this approach gives you a set of really tough questions to ask.

SETTLE ON ONE OR TWO TOP RUNNERS. *Then* get a demonstration, and see if your office staff likes the "look and feel" of the system. Demonstrations are not

particularly helpful in making a decision about a purchase. Most dealers start with a demonstration, which serves to confuse most staffs. A demonstration can be helpful, however, when you are ready to make a choice. You can ascertain the dealer's familiarity with the product by seeing how many fumbles are made while showing off the various features. In addition, your staff can vote on the ease of use of the keyboard, the user-friendliness of the screen layout, the speed of negotiating the various menus, and other such factors. You might want to see which, if any, systems are available with a graphical user interface. Do not give this too much importance, but, after all, good screen and keyboard design speeds up the work and reduces fatigue.

Step 7. Purchasing a System

CONSIDER FINANCING. Facing a five-figure invoice for a system can be intimidating, but if you can contract with a leasing agent, three figures a month seems a good deal better. Of course, you pay for peace of mind with finance charges, but you can easily budget a three-figure item against the expected rewards of lower accounts receivable, more complete capture of charges, quicker response to nonpayment from third parties, and faster turnaround on payments, especially with electronic billing and remittance.

DEALER MARK-UP ON HARDWARE SHOULD BE NEGOTIABLE. The dealer may feel that he can charge what the market will bear. If you know in advance the lowest available price on the items you need, you will then be in a position to bargain with the dealer on his profit. Do not expect to get close to mail-order prices. The dealer must make enough profit on the sale to pay his staff and provide for installation and set-up. I estimate that 20% over mail-order prices is fair. Many dealers charge double or more, leaving plenty of room for bargaining.

COME PREPARED WITH CATALOG PRICES. Catalogs are readily available from many mail-order houses. Micro Warehouse, Global, Computer Discount Warehouse, and Insight are good companies to check with before making the decision.

VISIT THE DISCOUNT STORES. As an alternative to studying the catalogs, you could visit discount super-markets like Comp USA, WalMart, Circuit City, and OfficeMax and check their prices for comparison.

Step 8. Agreeing to Terms: The Contract

BE SURE YOUR NOTES ARE WRITTEN INTO THE CONTRACT. This point cannot be overly emphasized. Dealers and users often disagree on what was said during an oral presentation, which can lead to much distress for both parties. *Write it down, confirm it with the dealer, and put it in the contract.*

AGREE ON MAINTENANCE COSTS. There are two kinds of maintenance agreement costs: hardware and software. Software costs are a bit more predictable because they involve dealer set-up, debugging, and solving inconsistencies with the operating system and with other programs running concurrently. Software costs should also include an automatic upgrade to the next version, when available (*see under* Step 5). Hardware costs are a bit less clear because they are a result of equipment failure. Make sure that your contract spells out who is going to find

and repair hardware problems and whether you have to pay additional charges for parts and labor after the warranty expires. Make sure that you understand how much supplies cost.

AGREE ON SUPPLIES AND EQUIPMENT. As a corollary to the above, be sure you understand what supplies and equipment the dealer provides and what mark-up is applied. Ribbons, forms, blank paper, and the like can be conveniently supplied if the price is right, but office-supply houses can compete for your business.

TRY TO MAKE THE CONTRACT FOR 1 YEAR WITH AN OPTION TO RENEW. Longer periods tie you to the same dealer for too long if the relationship is unsatisfactory. Shorter periods do not allow the dealer time to show you her or his qualities. A reasonable position is to agree to a 1-year contract with an option to renew.

Step 9. Installing and Using the System

The final step in the implementation of your new system is installation. This process has two steps: the actual setting up of hardware, peripheral devices, and related procedural concerns; and the training of all potential users to operate the software and equipment and to understand the procedures as well.

Hardware, Equipment Set-up, and Procedures

HARD DISK CLEAN-UPS AND ORGANIZATION. Insist that your dealer provide you with a full printed directory of all the files on the computer that are created and used by the practice management software.

You should also request an annotation for what each file or group of files does to enable you to make sure that all unused or temporary files generated during the installation process are erased. These leftover files can occupy millions of bytes of disk space unnecessarily. Make two copies of this printed file directory and store it in a safe place. Such documentation could prove invaluable if needed someday for system maintenance.

BACK-UPS AND ESCROW TAPES. Your dealer should provide you with tape back-up capability and enough tapes to run a routine back-up rotation. This process usually involves doing a full back-up at least once a day, with one set of tapes for each weekday, a weekly back-up, a monthly back-up, and a periodic back-up to be kept off-premises in case of catastrophe. Also, if you are going to be using clinical record modules on your computer, you can file a back-up tape with a lawyer once a month to be kept in escrow as proof that clinical data have not been altered after the fact in case of a lawsuit. *Do not neglect to make regular and complete back-ups of your data.*

CABLES. Be sure that the installer puts clearly written labels on both ends of all cables and on the sockets (except power and telephone lines), showing in clear English the destination of each. Do not be satisfied with arcane alphanumeric labels. Be sure that labels say, for example, "laser printer," "scanner," "modem," or "receptionist terminal." Also ensure that cables are all fastened to their sockets with screws or clips and that there are no sharp bends or kinks, especially near the insertion point. Make sure that wall plates are firmly fastened to studs or stable structures; often wall plates are just screwed into the drywall and can work loose after a few dozen inser-

tions. Remember that parallel printer cables may cause problems if they are longer than 5 to 10 feet.

TELEPHONE ACCESS AND SOFTWARE MAINTENANCE. The dealer has the option of setting up your system for outside access by telephone. Be sure that the dealer can do this, as it will save hours of downtime in case of a software error. Wherever the dealer has access to a modem and a telephone line, he or she can call into your system and provide software maintenance without having to drive to your office. If I were a dealer (and I have been), I would carry a laptop computer with a built-in modem for just this purpose.

POWER SOURCES AND SURGE PROTECTION. A surge protector is an inexpensive and essential piece of equipment for your new system. It is all too easy to simply plug your computer into a wall socket and assume that takes care of the power requirements. I wish it were so. If power were always exactly 110 to 130 volts, 60 cycles AC, it would be. Unfortunately, wall power varies from 0 to 5000 volts and from 0 to several million cycles in frequency.

If a truck runs into the power pole that holds your step-down transformer, the high-tension feeder line (5000 volts AC) can drop onto your input cable and send a surge of high voltage into every wall socket in your building. Circuit breakers are current driven, not voltage driven; so until the voltage has been acting on your equipment long enough (several milliseconds) to get a high current flowing, every input transistor and capacitor is subjected to a voltage at least ten times what is rated maximum, which can fry them very neatly. And if a circuit breaker fails to release, your power transformer can get red hot and burn out, not to mention start a fire. To protect your valuable equipment against unpredictable events in your power lines, you need a surge protector. This inexpensive device is voltage driven, and as soon as the surge hits the wall socket, the power is cut to your equipment with essentially no delay.

BLACKOUT-BROWNOUT PROTECTION. Next, you may wish to protect against brownouts and blackouts. For this purpose, you will need an uninterruptible power supply (UPS), essentially, a smart battery. Its circuitry is designed to monitor the line voltage, and when it drops below a safe level, 90 VAC or so, the UPS kicks in and converts its battery voltage to 110 VAC within milliseconds. Since the capacitors in your computer's power supply can hold a voltage for that long, you do not lose data not yet saved to disk. In addition, the UPS emits a loud signal, warning your staff to save what they are working on and shut down the system in the usual way before the battery runs down. Usually, a UPS has enough capacity to run a whole system for 10 to 20 minutes. Remember: *A UPS is not a substitute for a surge protector.* Most of them have some kind of surge protection built in, but a UPS may fail if a high enough voltage is applied to its input.

PROTECTION AGAINST UNAUTHORIZED USE. The best defense against unauthorized use of a computer is to encourage each operator to log out of his or her terminal when leaving the desk and to use a confidential password system for re-entry. Further, you may choose to issue each user a keyboard lock, which can work as simply as turning a cylinder key. Be warned, however, that these keys can often unlock more than one unit and are far from foolproof. A software lock is probably security enough. Screen blanker, or screen saver, programs—the ones that put fancy designs on your screen after a delay of a few minutes with no keys being pressed—such as After Dark, Intermission, and Iconfetti allow you to issue a password, without which the keyboard remains inoperative. Be aware, though, that simply turning the computer off and on could defeat the software lock.

ANTI-THEFT DEVICES. There are physical barriers to theft, such as cable locks for the boxes and keyboards, but these offer no protection against a determined thief wielding a bolt cutter. Such devices would, however, prevent casual pilferage.

The People behind the Terminals

TRAINING AND RETRAINING. Training people to use the program and keep up the equipment is an ever-present requirement with a complex management system. But you cannot always rely on your computer-trained employees to have all of the know-how all of the time. Employees leave and get sick. In addition, they forget what they have learned. To supplement the system manuals as an information source, agree on periodic retraining sessions with the dealer—it is worth the extra cost. You will be charged by the hour because no dealer can afford to contract for open-ended retraining after the system is up and running. The cost is amply justified, however, and I strongly urge that you do this.

CROSS-TRAINING. Back-up coverage among employees is important to have as a provision against vacations, illness, changes of job, and resignations. Make sure that more than one employee or kind of employee knows how to post payments, send bills, make appointments, run reports, and so forth. Often, any one of these duties may fall to another employee unexpectedly. If your office manager or bookkeeper, for example, becomes seriously ill, your receptionist should be able to step into the breach and run the financial aspects of the practice until the other employee returns. Make sure that the dealer cross-trains your whole staff, even the nurse and laboratory technician.

Employee Manuals: An Exercise in Implementation

One suggestion for putting your new computer system to work while familiarizing your employees with it is to use your new word processor (assuming this was part of your package) to create an elegant employee manual. We have done this, and it pays handsome dividends, especially when you have to bring a new or temporary employee up to speed. (Of course, you have the option of buying off-the-shelf software dedicated to designing a manual.)

I suggest including chapters on conditions of employment (hours, salary, fringe benefits, sick leave, overtime, and so forth); the duties of each kind of employee (do not forget small but important details such as who is responsible for locking up, setting alarms, or calling the answering service); how to handle common emergencies such as power outages, telephone problems, and computer crashes and less common emergencies like fire, windstorm, and flood; regulations and procedures pertaining to the use of the computer system; your practice-specific guidelines; and more. Do not forget to include a section on OSHA requirements. I have created an OSHA manual based on a copy of the law, which has focused our staff on the importance of complying with the regulations about matters such as training, labeling, cleaning, and protection.

Get each employee to help by being responsible for certain areas of information and making notes on her or his computer. These notes may then be assembled, edited, and incorporated into the manual as a means of helping temporary and new employees. If a full-fledged manual seems too ambitious at first, start with individual policy sheets on items like hours, duties, vacations, illnesses, and fringe benefits. Be as specific as possible about policies such as logging out of a terminal when leaving the work area. The computer can trace the person responsible for each entry or operation so that you can zero in on errors and malfeasance, but you can do this only if logging in and out is enforced rigidly. Attempting to write down your various computer policies and procedures forces you to be clear and knowledgeable about these important new concerns.

If the task of documenting office life sounds intimidating, break it down into separate information sheets or isolated paragraphs; this technique can make the goal of creating an employee manual a realistic and manageable one. Your staff can work on the manual in pieces, as time permits, and the outline feature of your word processor can help to structure the whole. Before you know it, the manual will be complete.

The implementation of your practice management system is an ongoing process, and a good place to start is by encouraging creative use of your new system while producing valuable materials for the entire office. Your practice management system itself will not ensure that your office runs smoothly and efficiently. However, such a system can be a powerful tool for managing the information flow necessary in a well-run practice.

2

MEDICAL RECORD SYSTEMS FOR OFFICE PRACTICE

Marc Overhage, MD, PhD; and Clement J. McDonald, MD, FACP

HOW CAN A COMPUTERIZED MEDICAL RECORD SYSTEM HELP ME IN MY PRACTICE?

If you have been to a medical computing meeting or have been following the arguments of the Institute of Medicine advocating the use of the computer-based patient record as an essential technology for health care, then you are already aware of the many benefits of a computer-stored medical record system. Computerized medical record systems offer the practitioner many advantages, including:

- Instant access to all of your patients' records from nearly anywhere

- Well-organized and well-presented data, directed toward the medical problem of immediate concern

- Flowsheets and graphs, generated instantly

- Back-to-work, insurance, disability, and other forms, produced immediately

- Automatic prescribing assistance that takes into account allergies, drug interactions, renal function, and cost

- Support for calculating physiologic parameters such as creatinine clearance rates, ideal body weight, and others

- Searching capability that identifies patients by any combination of clinical characteristics for research, management, or quality assurance purposes

- Reminders about preventive care, treatment guidelines, and patient recalls
- Online display of diagnostic images such as chest x-rays and electrocardiographic tracings.

All of this and more is possible. Each of the above capabilities has already been implemented in one or more practices or institutions.

Once all of a patient's information is available in a single electronic medical record (EMR), software can rearrange and present the data in various formats for different needs. For example, when referring a patient with a puzzling problem to an endocrinologist, the patient's test results to date, your progress notes, and other relevant data can all be combined to create a consultation-request letter. Or the computer could graph the blood glucose levels and overlay the glycosylated hemoglobin results, so you can illustrate to a patient what you mean by "good control."

Health care delivery has evolved away from isolated family physicians or general practitioners providing comprehensive services to patients. Complex, highly interactive teams of providers and ancillary personnel typify today's practice. Current EMR systems and telecommunications technology allow providers at one site or many sites to share a patient's EMR—a feat that is impossible with only a paper medical record. You may be at the hospital when a nurse at the office answers a patient's call. While on the telephone with the nurse, you can review the same patient information that the nurse is looking at, eliminating the need to ask for specific information from the chart. One outcome of this evolution is the need for a multiuser system.

Some evidence exists that applications embedded in EMRs can improve quality and lower the cost of care. For example, showing providers test costs, previous laboratory results, and patient-specific reminders or protocols can each have beneficial effects on the process or outcome of care. Completeness and legibility of electronic records also tend to be superior compared with traditional methods. The high-quality published studies of the value of EMRs, which assess the technology from different perspectives, generally show benefits.

Computerized Record Keeping: An Office Scenario

Mr. Dudley comes to see you for a scheduled visit after hospitalization for upper gastrointestinal bleeding. On the workstation in the examination room, you call up Mr. Dudley's electronic chart. The first screen provides a clinical abstract including the date of his hospitalization, the discharge diagnosis, and the procedures performed. It also states that Mr. Dudley visited the gastroenterologist last week for a follow-up endoscopy, although the summary report of that study is not yet available. In addition, the abstract includes data on hemoglobin measures taken while Mr. Dudley was in the hospital and on the drugs he received, including the doses. Next, you call up a screen containing a list of reminders: Mr. Dudley is due for colon cancer screening and should have a follow-up hemoglobin test. A template for a customized progress note already contains the patient's demographic information, which was loaded automatically, and his vital signs, which were entered earlier by your nurse.

During your visit with Mr. Dudley, you discuss his recent gastrointestinal bleed and his chronic hypertension problem, and you perform a focused physical examination. You edit items on templates that capture key features of the patient's problems in structured form. You also enter free text to expand on your observations and the patient's comments. Proposed orders from computer-based protocols suggest that you give Mr. Dudley cards to test for occult blood, run a complete blood count and liver-function tests (since he is receiving an H_2 blocker), and prescribe antibiotic therapy to treat the *Helicobacter pylori* infection, which grew from the gastroenterologist's biopsy specimen. From a menu, you select upper gastrointestinal bleeding as the primary visit diagnosis, accept the system's recommendations for triple antibiotic therapy, renew Mr. Dudley's antihypertensive therapy with a single keystroke, and confirm the order for a complete blood count. However, you cancel the order for liver-function tests because you anticipate only 10 more days of therapy with the H_2 blockers.

After sending an electronic request to your office assistant to schedule a return visit in 2 months, you sign the orders with your confidential password. The prescription is sent via electronic mail to Mr. Dudley's preferred pharmacy. You review the treat-ment plan with Mr. Dudley and provide him with an updated printout of his problem and medication lists. At the front desk, your office assistant schedules a follow-up appointment with Mr. Dudley and prints out a billing slip for him, which includes the appointment date and a bar-coded requisition for a complete blood count to be done in your office laboratory.

This picture is attractive but potentially misleading. Although the capability to do all of this exists today, it does not exist in a single commercially available software package. Before any of the current systems can provide even a subset of the services described here, a great deal of labor and planning must be devoted to various tasks, including transferring patient data into a computerized form.

WHAT TYPES OF ELECTRONIC MEDICAL RECORD SYSTEMS ARE AVAILABLE?

Three types of EMRs exist. The first type is an extension to an office management package that adds the capability to store and retrieve patients' clinical data along with their billing and other data. These systems integrate EMR modules within a specific practice management system. The second type is a program designed primarily for capturing clinical data. These programs can function independently, and many provide links to existing practice management systems. The distinction between this and the first type blurs in practice because most of the clinically oriented packages provide interfaces to office management systems to avoid the need to register the patient in two systems. The third type is the institutionally based medical record system, either community-based or associated with a local hospital or managed-care organization, which your office might be invited to share.

Extensions to office management packages closely integrate the patient's financial and clinical data, reducing the need for redundant data capture. Patient billing diagnoses, billable procedures performed, data from visits, and demographics are already being captured and can be used for both clinical and financial purposes. Clinically focused systems usually provide support for more detailed clinical data but, depending on their links with office management programs, may require redundant data entry. Using the third, or institutionally based, type of medical record system offers the advantage of someone else managing the system and worrying about linking to laboratories, pharmacies, and other sources of data.

Table 2-1. Patient Information Management Products Discussed

Product	Platform	Publisher or Manufacturer	Address	Phone and Fax Numbers, E-mail Address
ClinicaLogic 3.08 (DOS) Logician (Windows)	DOS, Windows	MedicaLogic	15400 N.W. Greenbrier Parkway Suite 400 Beaverton, OR 97006	Tel: 503-531-7000 Fax: 503-531-7001
Doctor's Office	Windows 3.11	PENKnowledge, Inc.	1075 13th Street South Birmingham, AL 35205	Tel: 205-934-3718 Fax: 205-975-6493 E-mail: bcouncil @penkno.com
MediMac 3.8	Macintosh	Healthcare Communications, Inc.	300 South 68th Street Suite 100 Lincoln, NE 68510	Tel: 402-489-0391 Fax: 402-489-6411
MediView	UNIX, AIX	Physician Computer Network, Inc.	1200 The American Road Morris Plains, NJ 07950	Tel: 201-490-3100 Fax: 201-490-3101
MedTrac 5.30	UNIX	Medicomp Systems, Inc.	14585 Avion Parkway Suite 1000 Chantilly, VA 22021	Tel: 703-803-8080
PAL/MED	DOS, UNIX, AIX, XENIX, Windows	Medical Synergies Corp.	4360 Chamblee Dunwoody Road Suite 400 Atlanta, GA 30341	Tel: 800-285-8602 Fax: 404-458-0319
Practice Partner, Patient Records 4.01	DOS, UNIX, Novell	Physician Micro Systems, Inc.	2033 Sixth Avenue Suite 707 Seattle, WA 98121	Tel: 206-441-8490 Fax: 206-441-8915

Electronic medical record programs of the first two types are briefly discussed below to illustrate various approaches; we included programs that are integrally linked to specific practice management systems as well as those that can be used as stand-alone medical records. We included some programs with a text/word-processing focus and others with a database focus. A list of the programs discussed in this section is given in Table 2-1. The reader can use this discussion as a starting point for identifying and evaluating potentially useful systems for practice.

Integrated EMR/Practice Management Systems

Practice Partner

The Patient Records component of Practice Partner is part of a series of integrated programs including appointment scheduling, billing, and a specialized word processing program. These modules can share patient information. Users navigate through the program via hierarchical menus, which experienced users can bypass via quick codes.

The Patient Records template for the patient's chart divides information into sections such as progress notes, x-rays, problem lists, diagnoses, medications, and laboratory data. Some sections consist entirely of free text; others, characterized as nontext, include structured lists or numeric or coded data, or both. However, free text can be partially coded by means of embedded "dot" codes. To identify an item as a major problem, for example, you enter ".MP:" followed by the problem name and, optionally, an ICD-9 code.

This dot-code data is exported to various parts of the system and can be used to selectively retrieve text. For example, coded information in a progress note can automatically update the problem list, health maintenance status, and allergies list; conversely, writing a prescription updates the progress note. The same dot-code approach can be used instead of computer forms to enter laboratory results into the fully structured (nontext) sections of the chart.

Several tools support data entry. The software comes with templates for 100 common problems and 50 physical examination variants. Users modify the templates to create a clinical note. The system also generates prescriptions and can check for drug interactions and allergies. In addition, patient-medication information sheets that translate prescription instructions into lay terms can be printed. User-configurable flow charts are available to display laboratory data. The DOS version of the program supports embedded graphics in the text portions of the chart.

Because the program treats nearly all data as text, little data-entry error checking occurs. A comprehensive query capability is provided but is limited by the lack of enforcement of a data dictionary. Because you can assign many different names to a problem such as diabetes—for example, "type II diabetes mellitus," "adult-onset diabetes," or "NIDDM"—the computer has trouble finding all patients with type II diabetes unless you consistently use the same name. This problem is an inherent issue in systems that allow users to enter key information in their own words. Forthcoming versions of Practice Partner are expected to help ensure consistency in naming clinical problems.

Practice Partner provides a health maintenance reminder system based on patient age and gender that enables you to define procedures to be done at specific time intervals. Health maintenance status can be updated through notations in the progress note or by appropriate data entry (for example, Papanicolaou or mammogram results).

MediMac

The clinical view portion of MediMac is another example of an EMR embedded in a comprehensive office management system. This system runs on an Apple Macintosh and can store and retrieve multimedia data, including images, sound, text, and data. Its Patient Information Matrix function lets you create spreadsheets that can contain any kind of patient data. You can create separate matrices for vital signs, diabetic flowsheets, and medication profiles. The system imposes no control over the values that you enter into the cells of the spreadsheets, and the records cannot be computer searched. MediMac does not provide for reminders or alerts.

The program fully exploits the strengths of the Macintosh system in terms of text and multimedia management and allows you to organize the data in useful ways. However, the current version's approach precludes achieving the full benefits available from an EMR. (The forthcoming version of MediMac will offer a more comprehensive EMR built on a database approach that provides search, and probably reminder, capabilities.)

MediView

MediView, available from Physician Computer Network, Inc., is a patient record system fully integrated into their practice management system called The Resident. The program supports the problem-oriented approach to medical record keeping and accepts textual, numeric, and coded data. You can define the list of data elements you want to store, their allowable values, and special verification checks to help ensure that reasonable values have been entered for the data element. MediView also provides extensive linkages between components of the record. For example, it links the problem list with diagnoses and treatments, laboratory results with orders, and so on. Progress notes are stored as free text, but many other elements are recorded as coded or numeric values. A useful feature of MediView is the ability to import and export text between the EMR and your favorite word processing program. This feature can facilitate functions such as writing letters on behalf of patients to consultants or others.

MediView has strong data-entry features. You can construct your own forms to match existing paper forms and greatly simplify data entry. The system imports data from laboratories, but only from facilities supporting Physician Computer Network's own exchange format. A full-featured query language allows retrieval both within and across patients on any coded or numeric data. Report formatting is flexible. A powerful protocol-writing function permits you to define reminders and clinical alerts. The program runs on IBM and IBM-compatible computers.

PAL/MED

Medical Synergies Corporation markets a product called PAL/MED—The Complete Medical Office System—which includes both financial applications and EMRs. The medical-records-only version is called PAL/MED Electronic Medical Record. Data in the medical records are organized into groups such as medications, problems, and subjective-objective-assessment-plan (S-O-A-P) notes. Clinical data such as laboratory results are stored as text without any input controls on the names of tests or their values, although the system does supply a suggested list of test abbreviations. The entry of medications is controlled by a dictionary of valid medications. This system has no query capabilities, but you can implement reminders scheduled for specific times, for example, every 6 months or when a patient becomes 50 years old. The physician must take the initiative to place a patient on a particular follow-up list, but once he or she is on such a list the computer does the rest of the follow-up work. Medical Synergies Corporation is releasing a graphical user interface for PAL/MED that will provide pen-input capability.

Independent EMR Systems

ClinicaLogic

ClinicaLogic is a DOS-based medical record system that can be integrated with existing practice management systems. ClinicaLogic organizes clinical data into categories such as diagnoses, notes, medications, allergies, and laboratory data. All data are stored as free text, which can be searched using an inquiry function. Templates for entering patient data can be customized when installing the software. Data can be entered using the template either by the physician or by transcription from handwritten or dictated instructions from the physician. Reminder and recall capabilities include notifying the physician about tests to be done at specified intervals based on age, gender, and diagnoses.

Optional modules are available. One module, LabLogic, enables direct uploading of laboratory results to ClinicaLogic. HealthLogic prints patient education handouts, and PharmacoLogic checks for drug interactions. Logician is the recently released Windows-based version of ClinicaLogic (Figure 2-1).

Figure 2-1. A summary screen from Logician, an electronic medical record keeping program for Windows from MedicaLogic.

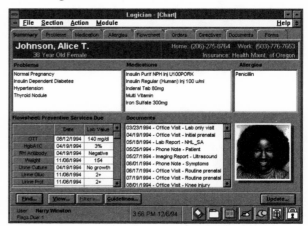

MedTrac

MedTrac was originally developed as a decision support program. Because such programs require extensive clinical data to support physicians' decisions, MedTrac evolved to include both data-entry and database capabilities; these latter functions have now become the primary focus of the program. MedTrac includes an extensive concept, or term, dictionary with several translations and synonyms for each concept. Data are organized hierarchically, and each observation is stored along with a visit identifier, date, concept code (a unique five-digit integer), and a coded result or free text. Data are entered using scanner sheets, user-defined "menus," or direct dictionary-entry mode, which enables you to pick terms that are as general or specific as desired. Other modes of entry include disease templates and step-by-step History of Present Illness (HPI) and Review of Systems (ROS) questionnaires. You may use a mouse or light pen, as well as the keyboard, when working with MedTrac. In addition, MedTrac lets you define a custom-marked sense form by printing questions and responses on a preprinted generic form that can later be completed and automatically scanned for results. Laboratory and other clinical data can be imported from external systems.

This system provides some support for storing images. It also has a full-featured query capability both within and across patients. Because MedTrac is based on a diagnostic expert system, powerful reminder and alert capabilities are available. All data are coded, and prose can be generated from the codes according to user-defined specifications. When creating prose, the system generates tables embedded within the prose from numeric data. MedTrac does not provide any office management functions, but it does provide bidirectional data exchange with one popular office practice management system, Medical Manager. If you use a different practice management system (*see* Chapter 1), MedTrac can create text files containing cross-justified International Classification of Diseases (ICD) and Current Procedural Terminology (CPT) codes which can be imported into your practice management system.

Doctor's Office

Doctor's Office was developed primarily as a data-capture system to be used by physicians for entering data during the course of routine clinical care. This system runs principally on pen-based computers. The patient information recorded in Doctor's Office can be organized in an integrated EMR with other data collected from various sources. Because of its initial focus, Doctor's Office does not now provide support for management of laboratory values and does not provide a query mechanism. Data are stored as coded entries that are entered into a series of linked spreadsheets (one for symptoms and diagnoses, one for medications, one for procedures, and so on) via hierarchical menus. A forthcoming version of the program will provide a more complete EMR.

HOW CAN I SUCCESSFULLY IMPLEMENT A COMPUTERIZED MEDICAL RECORD SYSTEM IN MY PRACTICE?

Your success in computerized management of some or all of the patient data in your practice depends critically on your understanding in two broad areas: the basic issues of data structure and source; and the logistics involved in entering and storing patient data in an EMR.

Structure and Sources of EMR Data

The advantages you see listed, or demonstrated, for EMRs are always on the output side: nice flow sheets, reminders, or instant output of the medical record content. But as you think about a medical record system, you have to remember that data input must always precede data output. Spontaneous generation of data within computers does not exist. All the work, frustration, and problems are related to input.

You should face the reality that once you have reviewed your options you still cannot store everything you want—not because it will cost too much to save it on disk but because it will cost too much to enter it into the computer. A completely paperless office is out of reach for most practitioners, especially those who receive large quantities of data from outside sources. Your goals, options, and potential payoffs are different depending on the size of your institution

(solo versus large group practice versus staff model health maintenance organization); the degree of integration between your practice and your hospital; and the type(s) of care you provide (for example, continuing, short-term consulting, acute or chronic problems). You must carefully weigh the benefits of a partial EMR against the inherent inefficiencies of maintaining both paper and electronic systems.

In general, the utility of your electronic patient data is enhanced by the extent to which the information is structured or coded, or both, because structure and coding permit your information to be automatically processed for various purposes. With fully coded records, the computer can more readily provide data for outcomes management, continuous quality improvement, automatic alerts and reminders about needed interventions, and so on. With increasing pressure from managed care and elsewhere for these functions, the need for structured data is likely to increase. This capability, however, comes at a price. Converting traditional handwritten or dictated notes into records with precise codes and rigid structure can require either extra (and expensive) coding steps or significantly different approaches to recording data (for example, marking check-boxes for history and physical items). Table 2-2 illustrates the complexity of the data-entry issue with EMRs by showing the types of information that you might choose to put into a medical record, where that information comes from, and whether or not it is structured.

When considering what information should be included in your medical record system, do not forget the information that predates the introduction of your computer system. If you have been in practice for awhile, all of your past records are in paper form. Entering all of your legacy data into the computer system is not practical, but you should consider backloading any old patient information that already exists in electronic form (for example, word processing files) as well as abstracting a minimum of information from the paper records of active patients (for example, important hospitalizations and principal diagnoses). This task might be done as part of a visit dictation as patients return after the computer system has been installed, but do not underestimate the magnitude of the endeavor. You will not be reimbursed for the extra time required, and it may require an extended period of time to complete the backloading for the bulk of your practice.

Considerable groundwork must be done before any of the above-described packages can be fully exploited. Much of this groundwork consists of building reference tables and including lists of laboratories, problems, procedures, and so on. Although this work is tedious, it is absolutely essential. In some instances, the reseller is willing to do some of this initial set-up work, but you should count on having to spend much time and effort to get things right.

Structured versus Unstructured Data

On the one hand, free text (as in a word processing document) is completely *unstructured*. You can say anything, in any phrasing, on any part of the page. No expectation exists that certain kinds of information (for example, the name of the referring doctor or the diagnoses) will be in a certain location on the page, will be recorded as a code, or will contain a phrase from a controlled vocabulary. *Structured* data, on the other hand, is best exemplified by a database record such as your billing transaction file: One field contains the charge code, another the date of the transaction, another the charge for the service. Each slot, or field, in the record has a predefined meaning, and the content is (usually) encoded in such a way that the computer can understand it—that is, the value is recorded as a number (for example, dates or dollars) or as a code (for example, patient identifiers or charge codes). The distinction between structured and unstructured data is not absolute because a database record could have a field containing free text from an uncontrolled vocabulary, and word processing documents have some embedded structure by convention. Nonetheless, database records are usually highly structured, and word processing documents are usually unstructured.

You will have many potential sources of unstructured data, including hospital discharge summaries, office visit notes, consultant notes, hospital operative notes, and radiology reports. We say "potential" because almost all of these reports are produced by word processing, meaning that an electronic version might be obtained. However, a lot of negotiating, a modest amount of management work, and perhaps some programming effort may be required to realize this potential. You should capture and store as much patient information from existing free-text information sources as is feasible to make the record as complete as possible.

However, available EMR programs, in general, cannot efficiently or accurately understand, interpret, or react to free-text data. Free-text records can be displayed on a computer terminal and standardized sections of a free-text document can be spliced together to make special reports. They are of (almost) no use for research, flowsheets, or graphs, nor are they helpful for guidelines, reminders, or patient recall. Information must be structured to serve these purposes.

When the source data is already electronically stored in a structured form (for example, lab results), you should attempt to preserve that structure in your system. Receiving the laboratory's reports as e-mail in your computer is easy, but it is just another word processing document and does not provide analyzable data. To preserve its structure, such information must be transmitted in a specific format. Whenever possible, you should obtain laboratory reports, for example, in a standard message format (*see under* Message Standards for Data Exchange), which has separate slots for a test identifier (a code), the date-time of the specimen, the value of the result, and so on. Most of the larger commercial laboratories and office system vendors support these formats.

Inside versus Outside Data

Table 2-2 shows the likely sources—inside versus outside—of the various elements of an EMR. Patient information imported from outside sources (for example, your consultants, the local hospital, or your commercial laboratory) generally presents more problems than the data you enter yourself. But once the link is set up, capturing large amounts of useful electronic data is inexpensively done, so it is worth the extra effort.

Table 2-2. Types and Sources of Patient Data

Type of Information	Source	Kind of Data
Hospital admission notes and discharge summaries	Outside	Free text
Consultants' reports	Outside	Free text
Procedure notes (for example, treadmill, sigmoidoscopy, bronchoscopy)	Inside or outside	Free text or structured
Referring physician's note	Outside	Free text
Demographics	Inside	Structured
Office laboratory instruments	Inside	Structured
Office electrocardiogram machine	Inside	Image and structured
Other office instruments (spirometry)	Inside	Structured
Nursing measurements (for example, vital signs, finger-stick glucose)	Inside	Structured
Questionnaire data (for example, patient completed history)	Inside	Structured
Visit diagnoses codes	Inside	Structured
Visit orders	Inside	Structured
Visit notes	Inside	Free text or structured
Sketches	Inside or outside	Image
Photographs	Inside	Image
Prescriptions	Inside	Structured
Outside laboratory (hospital or commercial)	Outside	Structured
Imaging study reports (radiology, ultrasound, computed tomography scans, mammography)	Inside or outside	Free text or structured

Word processing files from outside sources require a modicum of structure. Your computer must be able to find the patient identifier and the date and kind of report to file these data in any sensible way. The transcribers must agree to type the patient's name, number, and the date of the study in a standard place in the report or to mark these items with some special character. Your only other option is a manual review of each word processing document by someone who types in these three identifiers.

When you receive structured data from outside, each distinct clinical observation (for example, a serum glucose or hemoglobin level) is identified by a unique code assigned by the sender. Some results (for example, from a VDRL test for syphilis or a urine culture) may also be sent as codes. When you set up your system, you usually have to invest some effort to translate the senders' codes, and some ongoing effort is required to maintain the code alignment as new observation codes are added. You do not have to worry about this with unstructured reports. Some laboratory links to medical record systems are well developed, and some office practice medical record vendors have worked out automated approaches with the larger commercial laboratories.

For both structured and unstructured reports from outside, identifying the patient who was the subject of the report can be a problem because the patient identifier you use is usually different from the patient identifier the reporting service uses. There are two solutions. When you request services from an outside party, send along your patient identifier and work out an agreement for them to include the identifier in the electronic report. The message standards described below provide such a mechanism. The other approach is to enter the outside service's patient number in your patient registry and cross-index that number with yours. This approach might be preferred if you work closely with one large institution, such as a hospital. Social security numbers provide another possible link. Be sure that your medical record system has a workable approach to the patient identification problem if you want to capture outside sources of data.

Patient identification is not a problem for inside dictation as long as your medical record system provides transcription capability or a tight link to a word processor. The medical record system requests and verifies the patient identification, the date, and possibly much more structured information as part of the transcription step. Many of these programs go further: They provide a control over each part of the standard report (for example, chief complaint, the present illness, the past history). In this case, canned text and menus can assist the input. Some programs permit some mixing of coded and free-text responses.

With inside data, the problem of building dictionaries for structured information does *not* disappear. You still need to define terms. But you can probably build on the dictionary delivered with the system, and the work will be much less than translating an outside laboratory's dictionary into your system's dictionary.

Your visit notes and all the observations you make on the patient are inside data. Depending on the system you acquire, you have options for storing information as structured or unstructured data. The usual first temptation is to structure everything. Resist this temptation. The labor costs are roughly proportional to the amount of structuring you impose. Prescriptions, procedures, and some orders and nursing measurements (for example, blood pressure and diagnoses) are good candidates for full structuring. Parts of the initial history (for example, the review of system) and physical examination are additional candidates for structuring. If you are already using a multiple-choice questionnaire to obtain clinical information, these data are easily entered as structured input. Use a printed (preferably by computer) multiple-choice form on which office personnel can enter the data, or you can enter it yourself. If you choose to do much structuring, someone (you or an office person) must spend extra time doing it. Some structuring pays off well. You will probably save the time spent entering the first set of prescriptions in the computer by not having to rewrite prescriptions for maintenance drugs. Each office is different, and how much structuring you should do depends on the processes and problems that typify your office.

Do not forget that you can turn outside data into inside data. For example, you may want to dictate an abstract of the hospital discharge summary into your own office record if you have no way to import the discharge summaries electronically. You can do the same with key laboratory results as they arrive, or you could have your office staff enter them as structured data. (This technique seldom works, however, because the staff cannot keep up with the volume of data.)

Message Standards for Data Exchange

From the standpoint of office practitioners, two important message standards should be used when negotiating with information suppliers. These are ASTM E1238-94 (Standard Specifications for Transferring Clinical Observations between Independent Computer Systems, American Society for Testing and Materials; telephone: 215-299-5485) and HL7 Version 2.2 (Health Level Seven [an application protocol for electronic data exchange in healthcare environments]; telephone: 313-677-7777). The ASTM and HL7 formats are closely allied standards and are practically identical regarding the transmission of clinical observations.

Armed with an appreciation of issues related to the structure and source of EMR data, the next step is to consider the logistical issues.

Logistics of Entering and Storing EMR Data

Who should enter each kind of data? Prescription and order writing is best done by physicians; but it takes time, and some physicians may not be willing to do it. Different approaches and capabilities are required, depending upon the primary data-entry person. If clerks are entering the data, a paper intermediary document must be generated. As illustrated in Figure 2-2, the computer can be used to produce a stylized encounter form, upon which the physician jots visit notes; office personnel can then transcribe data from this form to the computer record.

Of the available ways for capturing information in an EMR, some of the technologies mentioned in the following sections are of interest but will likely enjoy more widespread use as they mature and come down in price.

Automatic Data Entry from Internal Devices

The data collection from some electronic data sources—for example, electrocardiographic tracings, blood pressure devices, and laboratory instruments—can be automated through specialized interfaces. Except for laboratory instruments, the interfacing is unlikely to be supplied by the office system vendor. If the volumes of these other types of data are large and desirable in electronic format, you should consider investing in the specialized interfaces.

Figure 2-2. A computer-generated patient encounter form. Note three valuable features: the preprinted patient-specific diagnosis list; a corresponding observation template; and, at bottom, a list of potentially indicated tests for the patient. The form also provides ample space for physician notes.

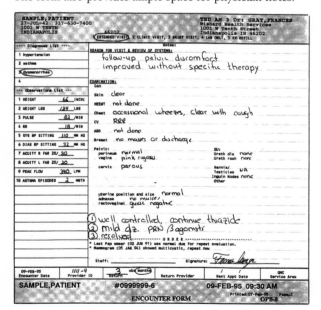

Automatic Data Entry from External Sources

As described earlier, you can automate the linkages to many laboratories. In addition, some hospitals are attempting to automate the data transfer between their administrative and clinical systems and their staff physicians. Registration, orders, and discharge summaries are obvious candidates for automatic transfer. You should be aware of the ASTM and HL7 message standards (*see under* Message Standards for Data Exchange) when negotiating with information suppliers. If you want to exchange data with commercial laboratories or hospitals, you should insist on one of these standards rather than on a proprietary interface for your clinical data.

Word Processing

Using a conventional keyboard and word processing program (with or without tools for structured data entry) is the most basic and readily accessible method for entering patient information. In fact, this technology is the mainstay of many EMR implementations, especially in smaller practices. With cooperation from your suppliers and some additional work on your part, your EMR might be able to capture your own dictation, hospital discharge summaries, consultant notes, and so forth.

Data Entry Using Bar Codes

Typing can be an inefficient way to enter information into a chart. The use of bar codes represents one approach to capturing the data more efficiently. Many opportunities exist to use bar codes for data input. Bar codes usually serve as adjuncts, not total solutions. The advantage of bar-code entry is that programs can accept these data with minimal user effort. The bar-code reader—a hand-held wand or gun that is swept over the bar-code label—sits between the keyboard and the computer terminal or PC and translates the bar codes into numbers or letters. To the computer, this information is indistinguishable from data typed in at the keyboard. The catch is that preprinted bar codes must be readily available and appropriately encoded.

Bar codes work wonderfully for tracking charts (the bar code containing the patient identification is preprinted on the chart folder), for entering supply charges (the bar code is printed on the supply package or a card attached to the supply), and for identifying specimens to an analyzing instrument (the bar code is printed on the specimen label). If your computer prints out a tailored encounter form for each patient, bar codes can also be used to speed entry of data from that form; you would print the patient's identification, the date, the encounter site, and the scheduled provider as bar codes on the encounter form. Since this kind of information must be entered as a preamble to entering clinical observations about the patient, "wanding" it in saves time.

Bar codes can also be used to enter detailed information. Typically, you print a "book" of answers to questions, such as "Dx this visit." A page contains one question and a list of possible answers printed out in both text and bar code. You enter your choices by wanding in the bar code corresponding to the answer that you want. However, this approach does not compete well with entering the same information directly onto a screen showing the same options, where information can be entered by typing a number or clicking on a box. So, except in special circumstances, using bar codes is not a good approach.

If you use bar codes, be careful about the kind of reader you purchase. The gun type of reader usually works better than the wand type because the accuracy of the latter depends upon the smoothness with which the wand is swept across the page. Also be aware that printers vary in their ability to print bar codes. Laser printers can print very accurate codes using a bar-code cartridge. Pin-feed printers produce less precise (but often functional) bar codes, but printing time goes up. This factor can be important in high-volume circumstances. The best bar codes are printed by specially designed printers such as the Intermec 4100. These printers use thermal-transfer labels which do not fade and which stick permanently, even when immersed in water.

Document Image Scanning

You can also scan in a page and store it as an electronic image much like a facsimile machine. This approach accepts and saves the content of all kinds of documents, including electrocardiographic tracings, handwritten notes, and preprinted forms. Data captured as an electronic image cannot be manipulated as characters in a word processing document. This approach has high storage requirements (30 000 to 50 000 bytes per page), and some manual labor is required to identify the patient, the date, and the type of the document. While not a desirable strategy for building an EMR, document scanning can serve as a useful adjunct when outside printed documents are needed in electronic format but other methods for electronically capturing this information are not practical.

Voice Recognition

A number of vendors offer voice-recognition systems, which translate spoken words to their typed equivalents. For example, if you say the word "cardiac," the voice understanding system converts that sound to the seven letters "cardiac." These systems have been used mostly to create reports of diagnostic study results (for example, those from endoscopy or radiology tests) and to record emergency room visit notes. Both semi-structured and free-text options are supported by the vendors. In the semi-structured mode, the clinician fills in blanks in sentence templates by speaking the appropriate phrases for each fill-in-the-blank in the template. The input is structured, but the output is often free text. The full-text mode acts like a transcriptionist and takes in all the words you say. However, voice understanding requires a pause...between...each...word. This can be tedious for type A personalities. The power and sophistication of commercial voice-recognition systems (medical and otherwise) are steadily increasing.

Optical Character Recognition (OCR)

Another option for external reports (and internal reports for which you have paper but no electronic copies) is to capture the text with a document scanner. Special character-recognition software enables a scanner to read a printed page and convert the characters on that page into text in a word processing document which the user may then edit and other-

wise manipulate. Some scanners are quite capable and can interpret standard-sized text fonts with accuracies of 99% or better. However, scanning documents can be labor intensive, especially in an office practice environment. It can take 20 to 30 seconds to scan and interpret each sheet, plus the time required to edit the scanner's misreads and to link the record to the right patient. Additional work may be required to capture drawings and some fonts. Moreover, preprinted forms and carbon copies pose special challenges. Handwriting recognition is generally not yet practical. For these reasons, we are hesitant to recommend the OCR approach.

Retaining Your Data

If you maintain a database of clinical information, we think you should plan to keep it forever. Permanent storage on disc is cheap. A billion bytes now costs less than $1000; that amount of space should last 5 to 10 years for an average office that stores all the text reports, treatments, diagnoses, and numerical observations for its patients. However, your system may have limits that preclude such long-term storage, so check with your potential vendors about possible software-based limits. For example, some system designs lead to slower access when files become larger, and some files have absolute limits on the number of records that are supported.

Protecting Confidentiality

As with other forms of patient information, confidentiality of EMR data must be carefully protected. General strategies for ensuring security and confidentiality of office records are discussed in Chapter 1. In addition to considerations inside your office, serious risks to the confidentiality of your system come from a telephone connection to the outside world. You must take special precautions to prevent unauthorized individuals from accessing your system. The three best methods are dialback, special password generators, and total encryption of the linkage. Dialback requires your computer to dial back to the number that has called it. Because it only allows dialback to preapproved numbers from which you call, this method practically eliminates unauthorized access. Unfortunately, it also adds considerable time to the linking process, so it is not always an attractive option.

Special password generators require that you carry a credit-card–sized device that generates passwords that are recognized by your computer. New passwords are generated every minute. You type in this password when you dial your computer. Because the password changes all the time, hackers can never guess the password by means of repeat dial-ins.

Total encryption is probably the most secure approach. Norton pcANYWHERE is a program that provides such encryptions. This method assumes that you are dialing in through a computer to a PC in your office. Since everything is encrypted (including the log-in sequence), the linkage is very secure.

Legality of Electronic Records

In the past, laws governing medical record issues did not have to deal with the complexities introduced by EMRs. The legal ramifications of paperless medical records, electronic signatures, and the like vary from state to state and are evolving. The value of EMRs, however, is increasingly recognized by state and federal legislators, and EMR-enabling regulations are emerging. Your state medical society, EMR vendors, and the Computer-based Patient Record Institute (CPRI) are three potential sources of additional information on this topic.

Successful Implementation in Practice

In the preceding chapter, Dr. Cushing offers a step-by-step guide to the implementation of a practice management system in the office. From defining one's needs to evaluating programs, systems, and dealers, this comprehensive approach may be applied to the implementation of an EMR system as well.

Summary of Issues

As you work through this system selection and implementation process, you need to keep in mind the various data input and output considerations discussed above. To summarize, these issues include:

- Data storage formats
- Data-entry support
- Report generation
- Data query capability
- Reminders
- Data exchange
- Compatibility with decision support systems
- Image handling.

For each of these issues, you must match your needs to the capabilities of an available system. Asking several key questions about the systems under consideration and keeping these needs in mind will help you find the right match.

DATA STORAGE FORMATS. Does the system support structured or unstructured data input (or both), and is a data dictionary used?

DATA-ENTRY SUPPORT. Are utilities that you might find helpful, such as templates, forms, graphical user interfaces, macros, and bar coding, provided to support data entry?

REPORT GENERATION. Is the system capable of creating the clinical reports you are likely to want, and are the report-generating capabilities flexible should your needs evolve?

DATA QUERY CAPABILITY. What mechanisms are provided to allow you to search for EMR data on one or many patients, and what components of the records are searchable?

REMINDERS. Does the program allow you to create a customized, automated reminder system driven by patient-specific data?

DATA EXCHANGE. Can data be automatically imported into the system from various external sources using standard message formats?

COMPATIBILITY WITH DECISION SUPPORT SYSTEMS. How easily can data in the record be interfaced with decision and practice support tools such as programs for drug interaction, prescription writing, drug interaction detection, diagnostic decision support, and patient education?

IMAGE HANDLING. Does the program support the capture and display of images, including electrocardiographic tracings and the like?

Experts mostly agree that at some point in the future all medical records will be created and managed electronically; their discussion and efforts focus on issues such as how and when this will happen. The challenge facing office-based practitioners is more immediate and personal; they must weight the costs and benefits of currently available systems to see whether now is an appropriate time to implement an EMR. We hope that the information presented in this chapter helps practitioners answer these questions appropriately and, for those who so choose, successfully implement a system.

3

MEDICAL LITERATURE MANAGEMENT

Lawrence Blonde, MD, FACP; K. Ann McKibbon, MLS;
Michael H. Zaroukian, MD, PhD, FACP; and Richard D. Guthrie, Jr., MD

This chapter consists of two major parts. The first addresses the subject of computer-based searching of the medical literature. We discuss the topic in general, as well as detailing information about online services and CD-ROM products available for literature searching. The second part, covering computer filing technology, discusses the use of the computer to organize your literature reprint and personal files. In a sense, the second part talks about how to deal with the fruits of your success with literature searching.

HOW CAN LITERATURE SEARCHING HELP ME IN MY PRACTICE?

Physicians are finding more and more that access to references from the medical literature can facilitate patient care, research, and administrative functions.

In this chapter, we show you how to get started in computer-based medical literature searching and provide tips to help you make the most of this important technology.

Keeping up with the medical literature is a daunting task. Given the current proliferation of biomedical literature, even a conscientious effort to read two articles every day still leaves physicians many hundreds of years behind in their reading after only 1 year.

Practitioners who are committed to keeping up, then, have to choose how and from what sources to obtain additional information when it is needed. Asking colleagues or simply going without complete answers is the most common response to specific information needs. However, referrals to or discussions with subspecialist colleagues are not always immediately available and may not yield answers that reflect current knowledge in the field. In addition, referrals are relatively expensive in the present climate of health care reform. Choosing not to seek additional information at all can lead to clinically

37

serious errors of commission and omission. Printed textbooks are often years out of date when published. To overcome some of the problems inherent in these approaches, physicians are increasingly turning to computer-assisted literature searching to help them meet their information needs.

Clinical practice produces information needs on a daily basis. Studies have noted the shortcomings of books and journals in solving clinical problems and have concluded that most of the practitioner's information needs may not be met during patient visits. Accessing, evaluating, and synthesizing scientific information is becoming increasingly important for practicing physicians who often feel overwhelmed by the volume of medical literature and guilty about their inability to keep current. This problem is most acute for those in generalist fields who must keep current in broad areas of expertise. Fortunately, we have MEDLINE, a mature and powerful computer-based resource for finding current published information for problem solving in clinical medicine.

What Is MEDLINE?

MEDLINE is a large database of citations to the medical literature created, maintained, and made available by the United States National Library of Medicine (NLM). MEDLINE is a computerized and expanded version of the printed *Index Medicus*, which grew from the reprint filing system of Dr. John Shaw Billings, an early Surgeon General of the U.S. Army. MEDLINE currently includes more than 7 million citations to the biomedical literature, dating back to 1966 and comprising more than 4000 jour-

nals. More than two thirds of the English-language citations contain abstracts.

MEDLINE is the NLM database that is used most often by clinicians and librarians. Other NLM databases include information (mostly citations or factual information) about the acquired immuno-deficiency syndrome (AIDS), cancer, chemical compounds, organizations, health planning and administration, ethics, and toxicology. These other NLM databases, together with MEDLINE, make up MEDLARS, the Medical Literature Analysis and Retrieval System. Also available through this system are listings of books and health-related audio-visual materials. Information on all of these databases is available from NLM and other suppliers of NLM database access.

Addressing immediate patient-related information needs is a major strength of MEDLINE searching. Physicians are increasingly using the results of MEDLINE searches not only in clinic and hospital settings, but also in referral letters, difficult or problematic patient situations ("you may not believe me, but as you can see from this article…"), training environments, committee and professional association work, and scholarly activities. MEDLINE is also showing up in the courtrooms. Verdicts have turned on the basis of MEDLINE printouts.

The Power of MEDLINE Searching: A Clinical Example

Your patient is a 65-year-old businessman. He has had non–insulin-dependent diabetes for many years and with proper diet and exercise has reduced his need for glyburide to a minimum. He has just been hospitalized with a myocardial infarction. Recovery has been routine but slower than anticipated. When you discuss his apparent depression, you find that he considers his "useful" life almost over. In his mind, the combination of diabetes and myocardial infarction seems like a death sentence. You know his prognosis is made worse by the diabetes, but you cannot quantify it either for yourself or for him. You tell your patient that you will find the evidence and bring it the next time you visit him in the hospital. That night you go to your computer and put the three major concepts—myocardial infarction, diabetes, and prognosis—into your searching program. The computer identifies 30 citations with information on these concepts that were published in the last 4 years. You elect to print out the ten most current citations with their abstracts, and one of the first out is a report of a study of patients with myocardial infarction. It has measured the influence of diabetes on long-term mortality. The 44-month mortality rate was 23% for patients without diabetes, which increased to 37% for patients with diabetes (Olander PR, Goff DC, Morrissey M, et al. The relation of diabetes to the severity of acute myocardial infarction and post-myocardial infarction survival in Mexican-Americans and non-Hispanic whites. The Corpus Christi Heart Project. Diabetes. 1994;43:897-902). You make a copy of this paper and give it to your patient. Although sobered by the 37% mortality rate, he begins to realize that his life can probably go on.

The search cost $2.22, and the time to do the search, scan the abstracts, and find and copy the article was approximately 30 minutes. A trip to the library would have taken longer. Textbooks often provide little information on outcomes when more than one disease is present. Compared with conventional literature searching using *Index Medicus* or other indexes, computer searching can provide fast, focused searches for needed medical references.

Do the Searches Yourself

Many physicians and other health professionals are starting and continuing to do their own searches; it can be fun and rewarding and, as the preceding scenario illustrates, has several advantages. If you know how to search and have the necessary computer equipment, you can use this tool anywhere without having to wait for or depend on anyone else. Results of librarian-completed searches are rarely available quickly or outside of office hours. Further, describing to a librarian exactly what you are looking for is often difficult. Sometimes even you do not know what you are looking for until you start to get your retrievals and can alter your search strategy accordingly. The ability to fine-tune your strategy during the search is likely to improve the results. In addition, once you have developed a successful search strategy, you can use it repeatedly to keep up-to-date on topics of ongoing interest.

Searching is not for every physician. Those who have no current or planned access to or interest in computer applications and those who are satisfied with their ability to keep current in their practices may not feel a need to search MEDLINE themselves. Most other physicians should be encouraged to try some MEDLINE searching. Benefits accrue even to the third of physicians who are trained to do MEDLINE searching and decide not to, for they continue to gain an appreciation of the literature, know what skills are involved in accessing it, and know how to interact better with librarians when requesting literature searches.

WHAT LITERATURE SEARCH SERVICES ARE CURRENTLY AVAILABLE?

The NLM produces MEDLINE and other MEDLARS databases at the National Institutes of Health in Bethesda, Maryland. As the issues of more than 4000 journals arrive at the NLM, they are read by experienced indexers (librarians and information specialists). Each article is then indexed with terms from a controlled vocabulary of key words (called Medical Subject Headings, or MeSH terms), and the citations (including authors, title, journal name, MeSH terms, and abstract, if available) are entered weekly into large mainframe computers. Understanding the process for indexing an article in MEDLINE can help searchers retrieve the greatest number of relevant citations and the fewest irrelevant ones.

Accessing MEDLINE: Online versus CD-ROM

The NLM provides access to its large collection of citations in several ways. First, you can access NLM's mainframe computers through a modem. (When you use your modem to connect with another computer across telephone lines, you are considered *online*.) The NLM also leases their databases to commercial and institutional database vendors. The commercial vendors provide access to MEDLINE and other MEDLARS databases and may, in addition, provide access to many other useful databases. Some institutions (for example, Georgetown University) lease the MEDLINE tapes from the NLM and provide local direct or dial-in access to MEDLINE for their affiliated personnel. The computer-support team from the hospital, university, or other institution with which you are affiliated can give you information on any networked MEDLINE options that are available to you.

After you sign up with an online database vendor, your online literature searching requires only a computer, a modem, an open telephone line, and telecommunications software (*see* Chapter 8). The online vendor may provide access to MEDLINE as well as other online databases. Most vendors provide the software that connects your computer to the host computer containing their database(s). Their software also generally facilitates search formulation and implementation. Accumulated charges are based primarily on the length of time you are connected to the host or the number of citations you retrieve, or both: The more you search, the higher your monthly charges.

The NLM also provides MEDLINE and its other databases to commercial firms who produce full or abbreviated CD-ROM versions of these databases.

Computer requirements for using the CD-ROM MEDLINE product are a CD-ROM drive, a computer that is fast enough to make searching efficient, a subscription to a product that provides the MEDLINE files on CD-ROM, and the necessary software to make them all work together. (A detailed discussion of CD-ROM usage is provided in Chapter 9.)

When deciding between online and CD-ROM searching systems, you have several factors to consider. Start-up costs and ongoing charges can differ substantially between the two options. Individual users who wish to access the complete MEDLINE database (containing citations from over 4000 journals dating back to 1966) will likely find the subscription costs too high for the set of CD-ROM discs needed. However, since the CD-ROM cost is fixed and lacks the ongoing use charges characteristic of online systems, groups of five or more searchers making regular use of the system may view a CD-ROM product as an economical choice. Individual users who are content to search a subset of the MEDLINE database—often referred to as "core" or "abridged" MEDLINE, containing 150 to 350 journals and spanning 3 to 4 years—may find this option more practical. Several such CD-ROM products are affordable and will probably meet most searching needs. Online searching systems become increasingly attractive when many databases are needed; when it is important to be able to search from multiple locations (for example, home, office, hospital, laboratory, hotels, airports, and automobiles); and when the most current and complete list of citations must be available.

GRATEFUL MED: An Exemplary MEDLINE Searching Program

To outline the process for obtaining relevant citations from MEDLINE, we chose one of the available search products to use as an illustration. While almost all of the currently available MEDLINE searching products are suitable for this purpose, GRATEFUL MED, developed by the NLM, was selected because it is one of the most widely used and fully developed of these specialty searching products. Many of the commercially available searching products have the same searching functions (as well as others) as GRATEFUL MED, but it is a facilitated online software program that is easy to learn and use, even for novices. GRATEFUL MED allows access to MEDLINE and the other MEDLARS databases, is inexpensive, entitles you to unlimited free periodic updates, includes a "How-To" tutorial program, and is available both for DOS-based and Apple Macintosh computers.

Clearly organized menus and a MeSH dictionary help you formulate your search questions before connecting to the NLM computer (the part that costs money). GRATEFUL MED then calls the NLM computer, conducts the search rapidly and efficiently, disconnects from the NLM computer, and analyzes, stores, or prints the results of your search for review at your leisure without additional cost. GRATEFUL MED can search by author, title words, text (abstract) words, MeSH terms, date or type of publication, journal, language, and other criteria, alone or in combination.

Table 3-1. Online Literature Searching Products Discussed

Product	Platform	Publisher or Manufacturer	Address	Phone and Fax Numbers, E-mail Address
CDP Colleague	DOS	CDP Technologies	333 Seventh Avenue New York, NY 10001	Tel: 800-950-2035 Fax: 212-563-3784
DialogLink	DOS, Windows	Knight-Ridder Information, Inc.	2440 El Camino Real Mountain View, CA 94040	Tel: 800-334-2564 Fax: 415-254-7070
GRATEFUL MED	DOS, Macintosh	National Technical Information Service	5285 Port Royal Road Springfield, VA 22161	Tel: 800-423-9255 Fax: 703-321-8547
PaperChase	DOS, Macintosh	Beth Israel Hospital of Harvard Medical School	Longwood Galleria 350 Longwood Avenue Boston, MA 02115	Tel: 800-722-2075 617-278-3900 Fax: 617-277-9792
Physicians' Online	Macintosh, Windows	Physicians' Online	560 White Plains Road Tarrytown, NY 10591	Tel: 800-332-0009 914-332-6100 Fax: 914-332-6445 E-mail: jsacks@PO.com

Other Searching Programs

Other vendor systems operate similarly to GRATE-FUL MED to retrieve bibliographic information from the NLM databases. These vendors use all or part of the NLM databases and provide their own searching "front-end." The product you choose should reflect your personal preferences in areas such as product costs, features, on-screen tutorials, and help in search formulation.

A selection of online and CD-ROM search products is given in the following sections. Table 3-1 contains a list of online search products, and Table 3-2 contains a list of vendors of CD-ROM products for literature searching. Most product and service vendors welcome questions and provide helpful and friendly assistance.

Online Products for Literature Searching

GRATEFUL MED

GRATEFUL MED permits user-friendly, online searching of the complete NLM databases. The program assists users in formulating searches and identifying appropriate search terms. This assistance includes mapping common words into their corresponding MeSH terms and recommending and defining useful MeSH terms for subsequent searches based on retrieved citations that you indicate are useful. The program allows users to formulate searches before going online, thereby reducing online charges.

GRATEFUL MED also offers a program feature called Loansome Doc, which allows the user to place an order electronically for a photocopy of any article referenced in MEDLINE. To use the Loansome Doc document-delivery system, health professionals contract with a library to make photocopies of desired articles to be held for them in the library, faxed to them within a few hours, or placed in the mail.

CDP Colleague

CDP Colleague (formerly BRS Colleague) is an easy-to-use yet powerful interface for searching MEDLINE and a host of other medical and general-interest databases. Proprietary software lets you search a combination of English-language as well as MeSH terms. A map function assists you in searching by mapping common search words into their corresponding MeSH terms.

CDP Colleague allows the user to store search strategies, which can then be reused at specified times to update reviews of specific topics, and also allows full-text retrieval from numerous periodicals and a variety of medical textbooks and nonmedical sources. This feature makes CDP Colleague particularly useful for the health professional who does not have ready access to a medical library. However, CDP Colleague does not provide the ability to formulate searches offline. CDP Colleague has a monthly minimum charge and substantial connect time and per-citation charges. Groups of ten or more users can obtain single accounts with significantly discounted rates.

PaperChase

PaperChase is a powerful, simple-to-use online service that allows searching of MEDLINE and Health Planning and Administration databases. PaperChase allows novice searchers to quickly and effectively begin to search and retrieve citations. The proprietary software lets you search using free text as well as MeSH terms. A map function assists in mapping common search words into their corresponding MeSH terms. PaperChase does not allow users to completely formulate the search before connecting, so that those who have poor typing skills or who do not carefully plan a search strategy before connecting can incur substantial charges. PaperChase has a fixed-price searching subscription available to groups of five or more users. For those with access to CompuServe, PaperChase is available on that service for an additional fee.

DialogLink

Knight-Ridder Information, Inc. (formerly Dialog Information Services), has a comprehensive collection of databases, covering an array of subjects in medicine, other sciences, technology, law, government, business, industry, general interest, humanities, and news. Examples include MEDLINE, *Morbidity and Mortality Weekly Report, The Washington Post, Consumer Reports,* and the *Occupational Health and Safety Letter.* DialogLink is a communications program that facilitates more efficient searching of all of the Knight-Ridder databases.

Table 3-2. Vendors of CD-ROM Literature Searching Products Discussed

Publisher or Manufacturer	Address	Phone and Fax Numbers
Aries Systems Corp.	200 Sutton Street North Andover, MA 01845	Tel: 508-975-7570 Fax: 508-975-3811
CDP Technologies	333 Seventh Avenue New York, NY 10001	Tel: 800-950-2035 Fax: 212-563-3784
Knight-Ridder Information, Inc.	2440 El Camino Real Mountain View, CA 94040	Tel: 800-334-2564 Fax: 415-254-7070
EBSCO Publishing	83 Pine Street Peabody, MA 01960	Tel: 800-653-2726 Fax: 508-535-8545
SilverPlatter Information, Inc.	100 River Ridge Drive Norwood, MA 02062	Tel: 800-343-0064 617-769-2599 Fax: 617-769-8763

Mastering the commands required to navigate the system can require a major time commitment. Knight-Ridder offers a computer-based tutorial and a full-day introductory seminar for new users. They also offer Knowledge Index, a lower-cost, after-hours information service with more limited search options.

Physicians' Online

This service provides physicians with free access to MEDLINE and other information resources, including Quick Medical Reference (QMR) and Physicians GenRX. It allows different search modes, including one that automatically translates plain English terms into effective search statements. Beginners may find it particularly easy to use, but it does not yet have some of the features of more robust services, such as the ability to save retrieved references in a format that allows them to be easily imported into bibliographic database managers. Pharmaceutical ads appear at the bottom of the screen.

Vendors of CD-ROM Literature Searching Products

SilverPlatter Information, Inc.

SilverPlatter provides a broad array of CD-ROM reference products on both Macintosh and PC platforms. Most of the offerings are networkable and support simultaneous use by multiple searchers.

CDP Technologies

CDP Technologies offers various MEDLINE databases on CD-ROM. They have several "turnkey" products, so that one purchases a bundled package of hardware, CD-ROM products, and interface software that can also support up to 20 simultaneous users, with local or remote access.

CDP Technologies has recently purchased BRS and has integrated BRS' online offerings with the CD-ROM products that CDP Technologies has traditionally offered. One likely outcome is the availability of more BRS databases on CD-ROM.

Knight-Ridder Information, Inc.

In addition to its role as a vendor of online databases, Knight-Ridder also provides both unabridged and subset MEDLINE access on CD-ROM with its product called Dialog OnDisc.

EBSCO Publishing

This vendor also provides both unabridged and subset MEDLINE access on CD-ROM with a product titled EBSCO.

Aries Systems Corporation

Aries' CD-ROM medical literature applications feature an innovative, probabilistic search engine that is particularly helpful for beginners. Figure 3-1 (top) shows the Aries Knowledge Finder search formulation screen, and Figure 3-1 (bottom) shows a screen with search results. Citations in Knowledge Finder are retrieved and displayed in order of descending relevance, with the first citations being those judged to have the highest likelihood of providing the information sought by the user. The software provides access to MeSH terms and also supports free text queries. True Boolean queries are not presently supported. Aries provides both complete MEDLINE access and several subset MEDLINE packages, which are available in both Macintosh and PC (Microsoft Windows only) formats.

Synoptic Resources on Diskette

A new group of electronic products does not, like the preceding, consist of programs for accessing or searching the NLM databases but rather consists of separate collections on diskette of abstracts from

Figure 3-1. Aries Knowledge Finder screens. Top. Screen for formulating a literature search. **Bottom.** Citations are retrieved according to the search formulation.

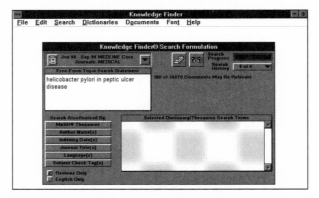

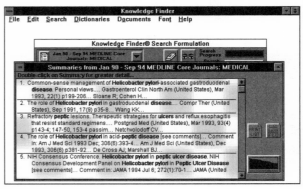

clinically useful journal articles. *ACP Journal Club,* for example, which is the American College of Physicians' (ACP) answer to the problem of reviewing the printed literature, has been digitized to facilitate further the task of rapidly identifying high-quality evidence on a topic of interest. It is currently available through ACP Online. ACP plans to release *ACP Journal Club* on diskette soon. Quick Scan Reviews (*see* Appendix, Chapter 3) is another example of such a resource. Several other electronic synoptic resources exist, each with its own criteria and methods for selecting journals and articles to abstract and for providing commentary on abstracted articles. Together with the database resources and literature-search programs we have been discussing in this chapter, these computer-based literature synopsis programs may further assist the practitioner in effective and efficient clinical problem solving.

HOW CAN I SUCCESSFULLY IMPLEMENT LITERATURE SEARCHING TECHNOLOGY IN MY PRACTICE?

Getting Ready To Access MEDLINE (and Other NLM Databases)

The first step is to determine which search product to implement. This decision should be driven by the characteristics of your anticipated searching activity, such as the databases that will be needed, the number of individuals who will need access, the frequency of searching, and the location(s) from which most of the searching will be done. Your decision should also be based on the characteristics of available literature-searching products. Consider the following points:

- Affordability (including initial cost and maintenance or upgrade costs)
- Ease of installation and use
- Type(s) of available help: context-sensitive; online; via telephone; tutorial program
- Concise and clear documentation
- Tools provided to aid selection of appropriate MeSH terms
- Ability to limit searches to specific languages, journal(s), publication types, and time periods
- Ability to retrieve any or all components of a citation (for example, title and abstract only)
- Functionality of the search engine
- Document-ordering capability to obtain the full-text article cited in the database
- Ability to import retrieved citations into various bibliographic database management programs
- Ongoing product enhancements (including their cost)
- Technical support (including cost, if any)
- DOS or Windows versus Macintosh compatibility.

As with most technology, some trade-off among cost, features, functionality, and ease of use is inevitable. You must consider the cost of the hardware (for example, modem versus CD-ROM drive, network versus single user) as well as the software and usage or subscription fees. You should also consider the products that nearby colleagues are using for their MEDLINE searching. Just as colleagues are useful for medical consultations, they may also be able to provide valuable advice on purchasing and implementing a literature-searching system. In addition, they may be able to help you expand your searching skills.

Some online vendors, including the NLM, have started providing special reduced rates for students and educators. Some also offer a "flat-fee" charge for unlimited searching over a period of time (typically 1 year). Flat-fee rates are beneficial for users who search frequently (usually two to five searches per week), remain online for long periods of time, or retrieve numerous references. One effective method for ACP members to use to get started with MEDLINE searching is to call the College at 800-523-1546 and ask for details of their flat-fee program ($200) through the NLM, which includes the GRATEFUL MED software, manuals, and computer tutorial, plus 1 year of unlimited MEDLINE searching. Local medical or hospital libraries are also good places to start. Librarians often offer courses and advice along with ongoing help and document delivery. If no local libraries exist, the NLM can be very helpful. If you are affiliated with a university medical center, you should check to see if they offer end-user searching services to affiliated staff.

These considerations, as well as the points on choosing between online and CD access to MEDLINE discussed earlier, should help you select a searching program to meet your needs.

Doing the Search: Getting Your Questions Answered

Searches of MEDLINE using MeSH terms are generally the fastest and most powerful. Searching for text words in titles and abstracts may seem easier at first, but this approach can miss many relevant citations. To retrieve the greatest number of relevant citations in a search, identify and use the proper MeSH term(s) for the subject(s) of interest. There are thousands of MeSH terms, and many search programs have utilities that help users identify appropriate terms. In GRATEFUL MED, for example, on the "Subject Line" of the "Input Your Search" screen, you can take your best guess at the proper term for the subject of interest by entering a word in ordinary language (Figure 3-2). If you then request the corresponding MeSH term, GRATEFUL MED responds by taking you to the area of the MeSH dictionary that best matches the word you entered (Figure 3-3), allowing you to select the best term for your search. Selecting the term while in the MeSH dictionary screen in GRATEFUL MED automatically incorporates it into your search without the need for retyping.

Occasionally, no MeSH term exists for a subject you wish to search, either because the subject is new or the MeSH terms are not specific enough. MeSH terms are updated regularly, but these modifications usually lag behind the early occurrences of new concepts in the literature. When a MeSH term for the subject you wish to search does not exist, then text-word searching may be necessary—searching programs can search for text words as well as MeSH terms contained in the citation.

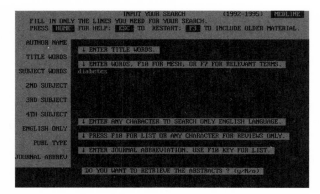

Figure 3-2. GRATEFUL MED's main search entry screen. A user has entered "diabetes" as the search subject.

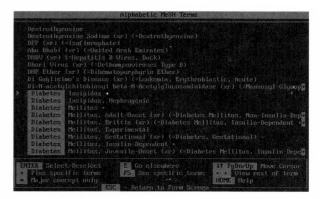

Figure 3-3. GRATEFUL MED's listing of alphabetic MeSH terms. The MeSH terms shown begin with the characters the user entered on the GRATEFUL MED main search screen (*see* Figure 3-2).

One reason MEDLINE searching is such a powerful tool is that it allows you to combine two or more MeSH terms or other parameters (for example, author, journal, text word) to define topic(s) by complex criteria and to retrieve relevant articles more fully, precisely, and effectively. To combine search terms, the Boolean operators "AND" and "OR" can be used in most searching products. Combining search terms with the Boolean operator "AND" results in the retrieval of only those citations containing all of the search terms in a single citation. Thus, the operator "AND" increases the precision of the search (fewer citations but more relevant). Combining terms with the Boolean operator "OR" results in the retrieval of all citations containing any of the terms in the citation. Thus, the operator "OR" increases the recall of the search (a more complete retrieval of relevant citations usually with more irrelevant citations).

Limiting Your Search to the Most Relevant Citations

A common difficulty among novice searchers is the retrieval of too many citations, many of which are irrelevant. One cause is the retrieval of many article citations in which the specified MeSH term was only a minor focus. For example, if you are interested in the prognosis of congestive heart failure in a certain class of patients and use the MeSH term "Congestive Heart Failure," you might retrieve an article that deals broadly with cardiac diseases, including congestive heart failure. In other words, the main point of the article was not the MeSH term(s) for which you were searching. Most MEDLINE searching programs allow you to eliminate such citations from your search retrieval. In GRATEFUL MED and several other searching programs, you can limit retrieval of citations to those that have as their main point of interest the MeSH term(s) you are searching for by preceding the MeSH term(s) with an asterisk ("*"). This can usually be done in the searching program at the time you select your MeSH terms. If you find that the number of retrieved citations seems too limited, or you retrieve no citations, try removing the "*" and run the search again.

Often, you will want to limit searches to retrieve citations only if they deal with human subjects or diseases in humans. Using the MeSH term "Human" excludes studies dealing solely with animals. You can similarly limit the retrieval citations to those studies involving certain age groups such as newborn infants or persons aged 80 or more years.

You may also wish to limit your retrieval of citations to certain types of clinical trials such as the classic randomized, doubled-blinded, placebo-controlled trial. MeSH terms are available to make this possible. For example, to retrieve citations describing randomized controlled trials, simply select the MeSH term "Randomized Controlled Trial." Most searching programs also allow you to further limit your search retrievals to "Reviews" of your subject, to "Guidelines," to English-language periodicals, or to certain selected journals.

You also have the option to retrieve with each citation a list of MeSH terms used to index that article. Although this option may make retrieving citations from online systems slightly more time consuming and expensive, it can enable you to find more relevant articles if your initial search resulted in only a few good citations. You can rerun your search with the MeSH terms used to index the on-target citations; this technique allows you to home in on the most relevant citations in the database. Retrieving MeSH terms associated with each citation also facilitates indexing of the citations, if you choose to import them into a personalized bibliographic management program.

Finally, most searching programs enable you to retrieve an article's abstract, when available. Abstracts are available for approximately 75% of the citations entered since 1975 but are not available for citations published earlier. Retrieving abstracts can add substantially to the time and expense of searching, unless you use an online system with a flat-rate charge or a CD-ROM–based system.

Saving Searches

Once you have created a search that successfully identifies useful articles, some systems allow you to save your search strategy and rerun it in an updated version of the database to identify new articles on a topic. For those who like to keep up on a particular subject by regularly searching the medical literature, this feature is particularly valuable; complicated searches do not have to be reformulated each time you want to search for new articles on your subject of interest. Various online and CD-ROM products provide this search-saving capacity.

Managing Your Information

Once you have learned to do computer-based literature searching, you may find that the end of one problem has taken you to the beginning of another: how to manage the new fund of data that so readily accumulates on your computer. Managing the store of bibliographic information is but a subset of the data management challenge, and here success for some lies in the implementation of an effective system for organizing all of your literature-reprint and personal files. Computer filing, like searching, is a specialized task with its own specialized tools—largely the bibliographic database management programs. We now turn our attention to the subject of organizing your information by using these programs.

HOW CAN COMPUTERIZED FILING TECHNOLOGY HELP ME IN MY PRACTICE?

In addition to managing bibliographic citations, filing systems help physicians to organize accumulated reports, reprints, notes, continuing medical education materials, correspondence, and other printed material. When used effectively, filing systems facilitate rapid retrieval of information collected throughout your professional career. These systems serve as lifelong learning resources.

Benefits of Computerized Filing Systems

The combination of powerful yet cost-effective computers and capable bibliographic database management software for both IBM-compatible and Macintosh computers has made computerized filing available to all physicians. Computerized filing technology should be considered by physicians who have a large or complex set of literature reprints or personal files, or both, requiring selective access.

As filing systems become larger and more complex, the benefits of computerization become more compelling. If you have more than 1000 articles, citations, or other items filed, computerized indexing provides the most efficient way to access your printed material. Computerized indexing and filing provide substantial cross-referencing abilities. The more cross-referencing, the greater the ability to retrieve specific documents. Cross-referencing within an electronic bibliographic management system also removes some of the decisions about where to file specific items in both electronic and print-based filing systems. For example, should a paper dealing with the evaluation and management of hypertension in women with diabetes during pregnancy be filed under diabetes, gestational diabetes, pregnancy, hypertension, or its first author? With a computerized system, a single electronic or paper copy can be filed in one location and accessed according to any of the above topics or others. Computerized filing also allows addition of your own index terms and keywords or annotations—you can put in your own comments about articles. Of course, computerized filing is not necessarily appropriate for small files or those where access is not a problem, because the investment in buying, learning, and using a new software package may not justify the benefit in these situations.

Most applications allow for direct downloading from bibliographic databases into preformed templates, eliminating the need to enter citations manually. Computerized filing facilitates the creation of printed bibliographies in various attractive and useful formats for conferences and publications. Computerization also facilitates the weeding or pruning of your files to maintain the currency of items in the collection. Pruning eliminates redundancy and helps maintain the number of stored items at a manageable level.

A complete master index of your files can be made easily, and you can readily identify all material of a given type (for example, literature citations and correspondence) within your database.

WHAT COMPUTERIZED FILING TECHNOLOGY PRODUCTS ARE AVAILABLE?

Computerized filing systems are *database management programs*. Indeed, you can purchase a generic database application (for example, dBASE, FoxPro, or 4th Dimension) and customize it to meet the needs of your bibliographic management and filing systems. However, several vendors have created dedicated bibliographic database managers with a host of important features, which, in our opinion, justify the cost of these programs.

Desired Characteristics of Filing Programs

Your personal filing system should have virtually unlimited potential for expansion and subcategorization, allow retrieval of filed material specifically and rapidly, and require a minimum of maintenance. The system should foster easy refiling, updating, and "pruning" (that is, removing blocks of outdated or unneeded material). A system should allow automated entering of references retrieved from online or CD-ROM databases; should support retrieval of references by complex search criteria, including support of Boolean operators; and should be able to identify incomplete references and duplicate citations.

The ability to save and reuse search strategies is a highly desirable feature of any filing system, and your program should also be able to save result sets of articles that meet particular search criteria (for example, all references that deal with hyperlipidemia, all references that deal with hypertension and type II diabetes, all references that have been discussed in *ACP Journal Club,* and so on). Many personal filing programs also have features useful for managing bibliographies and references within lecture handouts, manuscripts for publication, and similar documents. The program should work with most major word processors, extracting references from your master citation file by recognizing codes inserted into text, replacing the codes with properly formatted text citations, and generating a new bibliography file that can be merged with the text file and saved or printed in various journal formats. These features can be a tremendous time-saver for those who frequently write (and rewrite) and submit (and resubmit) manuscripts for publication.

A good system also allows users to copy selected files from one database to another. And in case you need to change your electronic filing system, you should be able to export your accumulated records so that they can be easily reloaded into a new system. Finally, the system should be accompanied by a clear and concise manual and a tutorial, along with context-sensitive help and menus to assist in navigating the system. And, of course, the program must be affordable.

Bibliographic Database Management Products

The products selected for discussion in this section are listed in Table 3-3.

dms4Cite

This full-featured bibliographic database manager is easy to use. Databases can contain up to 32 000 records, and the interface simplifies reference input, editing, searching, importing from commercial literature databases, and bibliography creation. Documents for which the program has inserted properly formatted citations and created a corresponding bibliography are write-protected so that any editing

requires a return to the original document for changes. Revised manuscripts can be generated by repeating the formatting process. The program is available only for DOS-based computers.

EndNote Plus

EndNote Plus offers versions for both DOS and Macintosh users. Databases in both types of computer can accommodate up to 32 000 records and have a reasonably friendly user interface and powerful search function. Importing from online or CD-ROM bibliographic databases requires the purchase of a separate companion program, EndLink.

Jeepers

This shareware program is available from various online information services such as CompuServe. Jeepers does not offer all of the features of the most comprehensive programs discussed here, but it is a good value and might be a good way for new users to experiment to determine if computerized filing with bibliographic database managers is an appropriate option for them.

Papyrus Bibliography System

Papyrus provides extensive bibliographic database management features in a single package at a reasonable price. Additionally, the sensible license agreement allows up to four distinct databases on any number of computers as long as they are under the direction of a single user. Databases can contain up

Table 3-3. Bibliographic Database Management Products Discussed

Product	Platform	Price*	Publisher or Manufacturer	Address	Phone and Fax Numbers, E-mail Address
dms4Cite	DOS	$$	Sidereal Technologies, Inc.	263 Center Avenue Westwood, NJ 07675	Tel: 201-666-6262 Fax: 201-666-8119 E-mail: jaegerr@acfcluster.nyu.edu
EndNote Plus (DOS 1.3, Mac 2.0)	DOS, Macintosh	$$	Niles and Associates	800 Jones Street Berkeley, CA 94710	Tel: 510-559-8592 Fax: 510-559-8683 E-mail: nilesinc@well.sf.ca.us
Papyrus Bibliography System	DOS, Windows, Macintosh planned	$$	Research Software Design	2718 S.W. Kelly Street Suite 181 Portland, OR 97201	Tel: 503-796-1368 Fax: 503-241-4260 E-mail: rsd@teleport.com
ProCite/Biblio-Link Package	DOS, Macintosh, Windows	$$	Personal Bibliographic Software, Inc.	P.O. Box 4250 Ann Arbor, MI 48106	Tel: 313-996-1580 Fax: 313-996-4672 E-mail: sales@pbsinc.com
Reference Manager	DOS, Macintosh, Windows	$$	Research Information Systems	2355 Camino Vida Roble Carlsbad, CA 92009	Tel: 619-438-5526 Fax: 619-438-5266 E-mail: risinfo@ris.risinc.com
RefSys and AutoBiblio	DOS, Macintosh	$$	Biosoft	P.O. Box 10938 Ferguson, MO 63135	Tel: 314-524-8029 Fax: 314-524-8129 E-mail: ab47@cityscape.co.uk

* $ = under $100; $$ = $101 to $500; $$$ = $501 to $1000. Prices are approximate at the time of printing.

to 2 million references, and the program has a user-friendly interface and many sophisticated features. Papyrus can screen for duplicate references and detect incomplete references. The large and modifiable bibliography format library accommodates almost all journal bibliographic requirements. At present, the program is only available for DOS computers, although the release of a Macintosh version of this excellent program is planned.

ProCite

ProCite combines comprehensive database storage and retrieval functions with a large record capacity and powerful search options. The program includes forms for many reference types and options for printing or exporting information to a word processor in multiple formats. ProCite's Authority List feature enhances both the speed and consistency of data entry for authors, journals, and indexing terms. Pop-up pick lists are available for each of these fields. Importing from online or CD-ROM bibliographic databases requires the purchase of a separate companion program, Biblio-Links. The options for the appearance of citation numbers in text are limited. Automatic numerical ordering, numerical range contraction, and spacing after commas are not supported [(20,5,21,22) versus (5,20,21,22) versus

5, 20–22)]. There are similar limitations to options for formatting authors cited in text and in bibliographies. Some other systems discussed in this section also have such limitations in their formatting capabilities. ProCite is available for both DOS and Macintosh users, and a Windows version is nearing release.

Reference Manager

This program, with versions for both DOS and Macintosh users, is comprehensive and easy to learn and use. One helpful feature is the ability to automatically scan reference titles and notes for keywords already in the database and append them to the reference. The program has some search limitations, and although it should accommodate the needs of most users, it requires the purchase of additional modules (Capture, Formats, and Splicer) to do so. Reference Manager also has some bibliographic formatting limitations.

RefSys and AutoBiblio

Biosoft publishes RefSys Super 3 for DOS and AutoBiblio 2 for the Macintosh. The programs provide most bibliographic database manager functions but have a single computer license restriction and a somewhat complicated installation process. Searches do not support the use of wild cards or the Boolean operator "OR." In-text citation is limited.

HOW CAN I SUCCESSFULLY IMPLEMENT COMPUTERIZED FILING TECHNOLOGY IN MY PRACTICE?

To help ensure that you reap maximal benefit from your filing system, you need to address several issues. To begin with, you should assess the anticipated value of the system in your practice and determine what items you want to file and how you will file them. How you assess the complexity of your needs plays a large part in purchasing and implementation decisions.

Assessing Your Needs

By answering the following questions, you will have a well-reasoned basis for deciding between simple and complex filing systems.

How much time will you devote to maintenance and use of files? Consider a computerized system if the time is significant.

What other resources are available (such as hospital or medical school libraries), and how convenient is your access to them? Computer filing can be a significant asset, even for physicians who have access to advanced hospital or medical school libraries. This is particularly true for physicians who computerize their personal files (correspondence, personal notes, and so forth) in addition to literature reprints.

What types of work and how many different functions (for example, patient care, teaching, research) will be supported by your files? The more types of items and functions to be supported by the filing system, the more computerization helps.

What is the size of your file—how many items will your system contain? The greater the number of items, the more likely that computerized filing will be advantageous.

How often will you use the files? If access to the files is needed on a daily basis, computerization should be considered.

How well do you know the material you will have in your file? The less familiar you are with it, the greater the benefit of computer options for filing.

How much information will be required when your file is queried? When you go to retrieve material from your file, will you need one or two articles on a topic, or everything on and around a topic? The greater the needs, the greater the benefit of computerization.

How much computing power do you have available? Computer hardware should not be a limitation to initiating a computerized filing system. The bibliographic database management programs run adequately on 386-based PCs; on the Macintosh, performance is best when using 68030-based Macs with at least 4 Mb of RAM.

Who Will Be Filing What?

Once you have assessed the likely benefit, several other issues should be considered in initiating and organizing a personal filing system. These issues center on the users and the types of material to be filed. For example, who will use the file? Purely personal files allow the use of subjective styles and terms. Departmental files, on the other hand, accessed by several individuals, require more control over inclusion criteria, filing strategies, and required retrieval capabilities.

What is the scope of the collection? What subjects will be included? Physicians may choose between a filing system purely for reference and a more diverse filing system. Consider which among the following types of material you will file:

- Just peer-reviewed literature contributions, *or*
- All literature of interest (including review articles, articles from "throw-away" journals, book chapters, and so on)
- Monographs
- References to chapters in textbooks
- Review articles
- Unpublished manuscripts and data sets
- Notes and handouts from course work, lectures, and so on
- Agenda books from meetings
- Government publications
- Pamphlets from associations and agencies
- Correspondence
- Patient write-ups

- Personal notes
- Pharmaceutical company materials
- Slides.

Filing Strategies

If you plan to file other professional material besides literature reprints, you must determine whether to file all material in one system or to create separate files for some categories of items such as literature reprints. In both approaches, physical items (for example, reprints, letters, and memos) are numbered sequentially and filed in numerical order from 1 to infinity. An electronic bibliographic database manager record is then created for each item to be filed. (If you prefer to keep entire journals and bind them for reference purposes, individual articles from those journals can be easily retrieved by using their citation in the database.)

The number assigned to the item is placed in a chosen field of the record. Other fields (author, title, date, abstract and/or annotation about the item, source, keywords, and so on) are completed as desired. This approach allows retrieval by both simple and complex (Boolean) criteria. For peer-reviewed literature reprints, data entry is most conveniently accomplished by importing citations retrieved from online or CD-ROM databases to your computerized file. This technique also allows inclusion of MeSH terms and the abstract, when available.

Lists that you create and store in your system for authors, source, and index terms can be used to speed data entry and control its accuracy and consistency.

Computerized Filing:
A Personal Approach

To exemplify an approach to computerized filing, this section briefly describes the system used by one of the authors (LB).

For more than a year, I have used a bibliographic database manager to organize my files, literature reprints, and all of my other professional and personal items that require filing and retrieval. Literature reprints are included with the other items, although I suspect that most people would file them separately. Each of the reprint records in the database has the term "Journal Article" included in the descriptor or keyword field. The database also stores a result set that includes all of the records with the Journal Article phrase so that I can limit certain searches to only literature reprint records.

As I become aware of new references that I wish to keep (for example, from attending our weekly journal club or perusing *Annals of Internal Medicine* or *The New England Journal of Medicine*), I (or my secretary) can manually enter the citation in the bibliographic database manager. I include a number of keywords in the descriptor field. I may choose to add personal annotations to the abstract field. The record number for the citation is written on the reprint, which is filed in numerical order in filing cabinets. If I wish to have the full MEDLINE citation, including the abstract and MeSH terms, I can later retrieve the citation with a GRATEFUL MED search and replace my manual entry with an entry imported from the search.

I have also used keywords to subcategorize some of the literature entries. Thus, I can quickly identify all of the articles discussed at our journal club or all of the key articles in an Endocrinology Section reprint file developed by me in collaboration with our endocrinology fellows.

If a staff physician, resident, or fellow wishes some references on a certain subject, I can quickly retrieve a number of citations from the file and print them out in an attractively formatted bibliography that includes abstracts and our own annotations. I can even provide them in alphabetical order of the journals included so that if someone has to go to the library to retrieve the papers, they can do so more efficiently. We can obviously pull the references by the record number from our files for review or photocopying. However, we do not allow anyone to leave our office with the original of any item in our files.

I have used the same approach to file a host of other document types. For instance, as correspondence comes across my desk, I attempt to deal with it initially. Often, however, the correspondence requests action that cannot be accomplished instantaneously or the correspondence is informational, and I think I will eventually have to refer to it. I then briefly make an entry into my filing system for the document: I will include the author, some information about the subject, the date, and keywords. If the document is an action item, I copy the title to my computerized to-do list along with the database record number so that when my computer reminds me of the task, it automatically prompts me to retrieve the document from the filing system. I have found that it is actually easier for me to do this than to tell a secretary how the item should be filed, since each entry takes only a few seconds.

In addition to correspondence, I have used the same filing system for agenda books and notes from committee meetings, boards of organizations, notes and handouts from continuing medical education programs, government publications (for example, National Institutes of Health Consensus Development Conferences), newsletters (if they contain something worth keeping for future reference), protocols for clinical trials and other research projects with which I am involved, and slides and handout materials for medical presentations that I prepare.

By including a date with each item, I can review entries for a certain date range to determine if the items are still worth retaining in the filing system. This pruning (which I admit to doing too infrequently) allows me to control the space requirements of the file.

Since I began this approach, I have dramatically reduced the misplacement of documents and the time required to attempt to locate them. I have found the benefits of my computerized filing to be well worth the time required for system maintenance.

4

DIAGNOSTIC DECISION SUPPORT

Blackford Middleton, MD, FACP; William M. Detmer, MD, FACP;
and Mark A. Musen, MD, PhD, FACP

. . . .

This chapter examines four commercially available diagnostic decision support (DDS) systems: DXplain, Iliad, Meditel, and Quick Medical Reference (QMR). These programs were developed explicitly to support the diagnostic process. Other electronic resources such as searching programs and CD-ROM textbooks may also be useful in diagnosis and are described elsewhere in this book.

HOW CAN DIAGNOSTIC DECISION SUPPORT TECHNOLOGY HELP ME IN MY PRACTICE?

To motivate the discussion, we first review the diagnostic problem in medicine and describe what types of questions DDS programs may be useful in

answering. Next, we give an overview of the ways in which knowledge may be represented in the programs and the techniques used for inference. Each program is then described in detail, with suggestions to help the reader determine if it is time to use such a program in practice. We end with recommendations for successfully incorporating a DDS system in the office or hospital setting.

Overview of the Diagnostic Problem

Recent analyses of information needs in clinical practice show that diagnostic difficulties are not uncommon. In addition, physicians sometimes have difficulty selecting and interpreting diagnostic tests used to evaluate their patients' clinical problems. Various computerized decision support systems have been developed to assist doctors in many aspects of medical decision making. Notwithstanding their increasing sophistication, however, DDS systems are not in routine use in practice today. A recent editorial review of the performance of the four systems described in this chapter resulted in a grade of "C" for computer-assisted diagnosis (*see* Appendix, Chapter 4).

Despite this unimpressive grade, if the use of DDS systems in medicine can reduce physician uncertainty, then they might decrease the number of diagnostic tests ordered and, in turn, one component of health care costs. Although DDS systems have been under development in research and other settings for decades, commercial systems have only been available for a few years. The relative novelty of these products; the fact that they have not been definitely shown to improve patient outcomes or satisfaction, physician satisfaction, or cost-effectiveness of care; and their relative complexity have limited the widespread dissemination of these powerful resources. Nonetheless, we believe that these products can play an important role in clinical practice.

Types of Questions for DDS Systems

When considering whether to use a DDS system in practice, you should first identify the types of questions that such a system might be able to answer. The systems are generally designed to perform case analysis in the traditional sense—that is, producing a differential diagnosis given a rich set of input findings. However, the systems are more often used as a *cognitive aid* to find answers to questions that are not readily found using conventional information resources such as textbooks or MEDLINE. These systems excel at giving the user insight into

relationships between a set of findings and possible explanatory diseases, as opposed to textbooks of medicine, which traditionally discuss individual diseases and their associated manifestations or findings. Using these programs, a physician may discover relationships between apparently unrelated findings that would be exceedingly difficult to discover by reading in a textbook about each of the diseases in which the finding may occur, even if she or he were aware of all the diseases in which the finding could occur. Relations discovered in this manner may remind the physician about hypotheses that were not considered initially.

Often, simple manipulation of the system's knowledge base, without performing a full case analysis, answers questions such as the following:

- What diseases should I consider given a particular finding (or small number of findings)?

- Is finding Y a typical or an atypical feature of disease X? Or can disease X produce finding Y?

- What is the best finding (or test) Y to "rule in" disease X? Or "rule out" disease X?

- What diseases may be caused by disease X? Or cause disease X? Or simply be associated with disease X?

If a more complex diagnostic dilemma presents itself and the user is willing to enter all the findings for a full case analysis, then a DDS system may assist the physician in identifying potential diagnoses he might not otherwise have considered, in critiquing a diagnosis already under consideration, or even in answering questions like those above in a full diagnostic analysis.

WHAT DIAGNOSTIC DECISION SUPPORT PRODUCTS ARE AVAILABLE NOW?

In this section we discuss four commercially available and better-known DDS programs to give the practitioner an overview of their design, strengths and weaknesses, and use in practice. We do not discuss programs under development in academic or research settings or those that have not been described and evaluated at least to some extent in the medical literature. To set the stage for discussion of the four programs, we first give an overview of knowledge representation and inference techniques used in these programs. Readers looking for a quick overview of how these programs can be used in practice may proceed directly to Methods of Use in Practice later in this chapter. However, before you actually begin using these programs in practice, understanding the concepts in this section will be valuable.

Knowledge Representation for DDS Systems

Current DDS systems use different methods to represent medical knowledge. Common to all these methods, however, is some representation of diagnoses and clinical findings (for example, signs, symptoms, and test results) and the relationships between them. For instance, a profile for streptococ-

cal pharyngitis might include symptoms such as fever and sore throat; signs such as elevated temperature, pharyngeal exudate, and cervical lymphadenopathy; and laboratory test results such as a positive rapid streptococcal antigen. When a disease and all of its potentially associated findings are listed together, a *disease profile* or *knowledge frame* is created. When all of the disease profiles and values describing the links between diseases and findings, between diseases and other diseases, and between findings and other findings are taken together, they constitute the *knowledge base* for the DDS system.

The values for the types of links described above may be a probability, a logical description of the relation, or a rule-of-thumb (heuristic) measure of strength of association. For example, for each finding-disease pair, these systems store some value that represents the degree of association between findings and diagnoses. In systems based on probability (for example, Iliad), sensitivity and specificity values for finding-disease pairs are used to record the strength of association. In other systems based on heuristic reasoning, ad hoc scales are used. For instance, QMR stores the data on the frequency that a finding is encountered in a particular disease as the *frequency weight,* which ranges in value from 1 (rarely occurs) to 5 (always occurs).

Beyond storing the likelihood of association between findings and diseases, some DDS systems also record causal, temporal, logical, and other types of relationships among diseases. For instance, QMR identifies diseases that cause other diseases (for example, Crohn disease causing enteropathic arthritis) with causal links. Similarly, QMR codes with temporal links those diseases that may occur before other diseases (for example, acute viral hepatitis preceding chronic active hepatitis). Finally, QMR codes with other links diseases that predispose to other diseases or diseases that coincide with other diseases. When these relationships are encoded in the knowledge base of a DDS system, they can help these programs to serve as useful adjuncts in the diagnostic process.

Inference Methods for DDS Systems

Given a scheme for knowledge representation as described above, DDS systems may use various methods to infer a differential diagnosis from a given input set of findings. The knowledge base forms the corpus of medical knowledge that is used by the *inference engine* in the DDS system to produce output such as a differential diagnosis. The inference engine is the set of tools and techniques programmed into the computer to analyze the input findings and determine plausible hypotheses given the information programmed in the knowledge base. Theoretically, an inference engine may be used with different knowledge bases, and vice versa. However, such interchangeability is not possible with current commercial systems.

For example, a hand calculator has an inference engine in it that knows how to do simple arithmetic. When asked to add 4 plus 5, the machine calculates the answer using the programming within it. Alternatively, a different inference engine—for example, an abacus—may be given the same problem and solve it in a different manner. Similarly, the DDS systems being considered here use various techniques to combine and weight evidence from input findings and arrive at a plausible differential. The simplest approach may use an algorithm that says "if findings a, b, c, and d are present, then disease 1 exists" (or is offered as the diagnosis). Such a simple approach does not allow the user to appreciate the likelihood of a disease, given a set of findings, or to contrast the strength of association between findings and a disease.

An alternate approach is to define a heuristic or associational reasoning method which may attempt to emulate human reasoning to a certain degree. Two of the programs described in this chapter use heuristic techniques to weight and combine evidence to produce a plausible differential diagnosis. QMR in the analysis mode, for example, attempts to determine the weight of the evidence for a diagnosis roughly by adding the weights of findings input as present; subtracting the weight of the evidence against the diagnosis based on findings expected to be present (identified in the disease profile in the knowledge base) but input as absent; and assessing a penalty for findings input as present but not explained by the hypothesized diagnosis. In this manner, the program attempts to emulate the hypothetico-deductive approach physicians are taught in medical school.

Lastly, Bayes' theorem may be used when the relationships between elements of the knowledge base are described probabilistically. Difficulties arise in this method, however, in arriving at the probability figures in the knowledge base and, computationally, in applying Bayes' theorem to real-world problems like medical diagnosis. Use of Bayesian techniques typically requires assuming that all of the diseases in the knowledge base are mutually exclusive and exhaustive. That is, they may not co-occur, and taken together they describe all possible diseases. In addition, the assumption of conditional independence of findings given a disease is typically made to facilitate assessment of the probabilities and the Bayesian calculations. This assumption states that the presence of one finding given a disease does not make the presence of another more likely, which often runs contrary to clinical intuition. An example of the difficulties with this assumption are discussed in more detail below. Other assumptions may be made to simplify the probability assessment and inference calculations, but they are beyond the scope of this chapter.

Four Commercially Available DDS Systems

DXplain

DXplain is a DDS system developed at Massachusetts General Hospital in the 1980s. The main purpose of DXplain is to generate a list of diagnostic hypotheses from a group of clinical findings. Users enter clinical terms into a command-line interface and receive a differential diagnosis ranked by likelihood. In addition, users can explore the relationships between diseases and findings by browsing through the knowledge base.

Representation of Medical Knowledge

DXplain's knowledge base is derived from information in the American Medical Association's *Current Medical Information and Terminology (CMIT)*. Currently, DXplain represents information on approximately 2000 diseases, 4500 clinical findings, and 92 000 inter-relationships. A disease profile consists of a set of clinical findings that appears in *CMIT* and that the developers have decided is relevant.

For each finding listed for a disease, three attributes are stored: term frequency, term evoking strength, and term importance. These attributes are derived from similar attributes in the QMR knowledge base. *Term frequency* measures how often a finding occurs in a disease and is roughly equivalent to the concept of sensitivity. Findings are rated on a scale from 1 (never occurs) to 7 (always occurs). *Term evoking strength* is how strongly the finding supports the diagnosis of the disease and is roughly equivalent to the concept of positive predictive value, or the chance of disease given the presence of a finding. Findings are rated on a scale from 1 (rules out disease) to 9 (disease must always be considered). Finally, *term importance* measures how consequential the finding is. A high term importance is given to findings that can be identified with high reliability or are rarely found in healthy persons. Findings with high term importance should be explained by some disease within the differential diagnosis.

In addition to storing attributes that define the relationships between findings and diseases, DXplain also stores information on the diseases themselves. First, DXplain stores a representation of *disease prevalence,* or the chance that the disease is present in the general population. DXplain does not store this entity as a probability, but instead as a category: *common, rare,* or *very rare.* In addition, DXplain stores the *disease importance,* or how consequential the disease is. Diseases that are fatal if untreated and that have an effective therapy are rated highest in this 5-point scale, while diseases that are inconsequential are given the lowest rating.

Inference Techniques

DXplain generates a differential diagnosis from a list of findings by first evaluating the term importance and term evoking strength of each finding-diagnosis pair and then calculating a summary score for each disease. A disease score is most influenced by positive findings that have high term evoking strength. Findings with intermediate evoking strengths and high term importance contribute moderately to the summary score. After DXplain evaluates each clinical finding, it displays the highest-ranked diagnoses divided into "common" diseases and "rare" or "very rare" diseases.

Use of DXplain in Practice

DXplain can be used in two ways: for *case analysis* or for browsing the knowledge base. For case analysis, the user enters clinical findings by typing terms into the command-line interface. Because DXplain has a rich synonym dictionary, most medical terms entered into the program will map to a finding stored in the knowledge base. Once the desired clinical findings are entered, a ranked differential diagnosis can be quickly generated. Users can then ask DXplain to

explain why a particular diagnosis is on the differential. DXplain shows the observed findings that support the diagnosis, findings that would support the diagnosis if present, as well as findings that make the diagnosis less likely. DXplain can also query the user for more clinical information to help narrow the differential diagnosis.

For *browsing,* DXplain can also be used as an electronic textbook. Users can view disease profiles (Figure 4-1), obtain relevant literature citations for a particular diagnosis, or view diseases that contain a finding or group of findings.

Figure 4-1. A portion of the acute appendicitis disease profile from DXplain.

APPENDICITIS, ACUTE (Very Common)

ETIOLOGY
Focal obstruction of appendicial lumen due to lymphoid hyperplasia, adhesions, fecaliths, foreign bodies, intestinal parasites; distention of lumen increasing pressure within organ; virulent bacteria converting mucus into pus.

ASSOCIATED FINDINGS AND CONDITIONS
USUALLY: ileus.
SOMETIMES: male; intestinal perforation.
RARELY: peritonitis.
MAKE DIAGNOSIS LESS LIKELY: appendectomy past.

SYMPTOMS
USUALLY: abdominal pain, right lower quadrant; anorexia; abdominal pain.
SOMETIMES: nausea; vomiting; abdominal pain, crampy; constipation; chills; movement pain; sudden onset of symptoms; acute; abdominal pain, periumbilical; epigastric abdominal pain; dysuria.
RARELY: abdominal pain, right upper quadrant; abdominal pain radiating to back; flank pain; groin pain.
MAKE DIAGNOSIS LESS LIKELY: diarrhea; appetite increase.

Iliad

Iliad is a DDS system initially developed at the Latter-Day Saints Hospital in Salt Lake City, Utah, in the 1980s. It uses a modification of Bayes' theorem as the basis for generating a differential diagnosis. Iliad can be used to analyze a clinical case, critique a diagnosis, simulate a clinical case, or browse through the knowledge base. In case-analysis mode, users enter findings into a graphical user interface and receive a differential diagnosis ranked by likelihood.

Representation of Medical Knowledge

In contrast to the other systems mentioned in this chapter, Iliad stores knowledge about medicine in the form of probabilities. An Iliad disease profile consists of the disease's prevalence together with the sensitivities and specificities of all clinical findings that are found in the disease (Figure 4-2). For instance, Iliad stores for the diagnosis "community-acquired pneumonia" a prevalence of 7/1000 for an outpatient population and symptoms such as "dyspnea at rest with recent onset" with a sensitivity of 30% and specificity of 95%.

The Iliad knowledge base is derived from two sources. First, prevalence and some sensitivity-specificity data are collected from the HELP system, a large clinical information system and database also developed at Latter-Day Saints Hospital. Second, groups of experts meet with the developers on a regular basis and review data from both the HELP system and the medical literature. Working by consensus, the group decides which clinical findings should be included in a disease profile as well as what

sensitivity and specificity numbers should be used. Currently, Iliad stores data on approximately 960 diseases and 11 900 clinical findings.

One of the problems with a Bayesian system for a large domain such as internal medicine is that traditional Bayesian systems require clinical findings to be *conditionally independent* of each other—that is, for a given disease, the chance that one finding is present should not influence the chance that another finding is present. In internal medicine, however, clinical findings are often not conditionally independent. For instance, in liver disease the aspartate aminotransferase (AST) and alanine aminotransferase (ALT) tests are not conditionally independent; the presence of an elevated AST level in a patient with liver disease

Figure 4-2. A portion of the pneumonia disease profile from Iliad.

FINDINGS:	●Status ●Cost	●TPR ●FPR	●LR+ ●LR-
●Lung consolidation by CXR		.50 .01	50.0 (1.98)
if True			
-- or --			
●Diffuse bilateral consolidation by CXR		.10 .002	50.0 (1.11)
-- or --			
●CXR pattern of pneumonia		.98 .02	49.0 (49.0)
-- or --			
●Lung consolidation by PE		.80 .02	40.0 (4.90)
●Acute Productive Cough		.97 .02	48.5 (32.6)
-- or --			
History of present illness: cough		.97 .10	9.70 (30.0)
Sputum gram stain shows gram positive intracellular diplococci	$32	.60 .02	30.0 (2.45)
-- or --			
Sputum gram stain shows gram positive bacteria	$32	.75 .40	1.87 (2.40)
-- or --			
Routine Sputum culture grows pneumococcus	$53	.60 .40	1.50 (1.50)
-- or --			
Sputum gram stain shows gram negative bacteria	$32	.75 .40	1.87 (2.40)

●Prevalence:7 in 1,000 for statistics in "NAMCS outpatient" apriori table.
●Posterior Probability: 0.0

Pneumonia

<- Bayes/Boolean Calculator

increases the chance that the ALT level is elevated. When conditionally dependent findings are represented in a traditional Bayesian system and all dependent findings are present in a particular case, the likelihood of a disease will be overestimated because the system overcounts the influence of findings that are manifestations of the same internal state.

Iliad attempts to circumvent this problem of conditional dependence by clustering all conditionally dependent findings and treating this cluster as one finding. Thus, when more than one conditionally dependent finding is present, the influence of those findings is counted only once. Iliad clusters conditionally dependent findings in what are called Boolean frames. *Boolean frames* define which combinations of conditionally dependent findings make the cluster true. For instance, Iliad represents the cluster "lung consolidation by physical examination" by the findings A) "dullness to percussion," B) "bronchial breath sounds," C) "egophony," D) "increased vocal fremitus," E) "crackles," and F) "whispered pectoriloquy." The cluster is considered true if A or B is true and two of C, D, E, and F are true. Iliad stores a sensitivity and specificity for the cluster "lung consolidation by physical examination."

Inference Techniques

Iliad uses a modification of Bayes' theorem to calculate the probability that a patient has a particular disease given the presence of some clinical findings. Using sensitivity and specificity numbers, Iliad first calculates likelihood ratios, both positive (LR+) and negative (LR−). After converting the pretest probability to pretest odds, Iliad uses the odds-likelihood version of Bayes' theorem to calculate the post-test odds of disease.

When a user enters a finding, Iliad first searches for all diseases that contain that finding and then updates the probability of each of those diseases. For example, when a user begins a case by entering the symptom "chest pain," Iliad searches for all diseases that contain that symptom and updates the probability of each disease. For the disease "stable angina," Iliad has the prevalence listed as 3/100 (odds 3 in 97) in an outpatient population and the LR+ as 5. Iliad then updates the probability of stable angina accordingly.

After calculating the post-test probability for each disease with this finding, Iliad then displays the differential diagnosis in order of likelihood. As new findings are added, Iliad updates the probabilities in a similar fashion.

Use of Iliad in Practice

Iliad has four modes of operation: consultation, critique, simulation, and browse. In the consultation mode, users enter findings, and the system provides a list of possible diagnoses ranked by probability. Users can either enter findings as free text (which must be mapped to a finding in the knowledge base) or choose from a menu of findings organized by assessment category (for example, history of present illness, past medical history, or physical examination). In critique mode, users enter findings and then assert a diagnosis; Iliad critiques that diagnosis by pointing out findings that support or detract from the chosen diagnosis. In simulation mode, users are presented with a case and are required to ask questions to arrive at a diagnosis. A simulation can be generated randomly from all the diagnoses in the knowledge base or can be generated from a list of diseases that a medical school instructor determines to be important for a student to learn. A user's interaction with the simulator can be scored and captured in a log file, allowing instructors to evaluate students' performance. Finally, in browse mode, users can look through the knowledge base, examining disease profiles and exploring relationships between findings and diseases.

Iliad also includes sample color images of some clinical findings, relevant citations and summaries from Mosby's *Yearbook of Medicine,* and treatment suggestions for all diseases in the knowledge base. Treatment suggestions and alternatives are derived from expert opinion.

Meditel Adult Diagnostic System

This DDS program was developed by Herbert S. Waxman, MD, and William E. Worley, MD. It is a descendant of the Meditel Pediatric System, which was developed in the 1970s to assist in the diagnosis of clinically challenging pediatric cases. The version for adult patients seeks to help clinicians in the diagnosis of systemic diseases—most localized conditions are not included. Unlike the other systems mentioned, this program is designed exclusively for diagnosis: No mechanism is in place to browse the knowledge base. Users enter findings by either choosing from a hierarchical menu or entering a three-digit code; free-text entry is not possible. Once findings are entered, a differential diagnosis can be generated (Figure 4-3). Users can then identify

Figure 4-3. A differential diagnosis generated by Meditel for several entered findings.

```
02-11-1995   11:12:32

MEDITEL (R) COMPUTER ASSISTED DIAGNOSIS
            ADULT DIAGNOSTIC SYSTEM   V-3.0
COPYRIGHT (C) MEDITEL, INC. 1988-1995


CAUTION:      THERE CAN BE NO ASSURANCE OR GUARANTEE THAT
              THE PATIENT'S DIAGNOSIS IS INCLUDED IN THIS REPORT.
              THE PHYSICIAN SHOULD CONSIDER HIS OR HER OWN
              LIST OF POSSIBLE DIAGNOSES ALONG WITH THE MEDI-
              TEL LIST. ALSO, NO SUGGESTED TEST OR PROCEDURE
              SHOULD BE CARRIED OUT UNLESS, IN THE PHYSICIAN'S
              JUDGMENT, ITS RISK IS JUSTIFIED.

PHYSICIAN'S ID: S. Dawson, M.D.

PATIENT'S ID: Record # 24856

SEX: FEMALE   AGE OF ONSET OF FINDINGS:  37 YEARS

***FINDINGS ENTERED***

      FEVER
      PETECHIAE; PURPURA; HEMATOMA (SKIN)
      CONFUSION; DELIRIUM
      HYPERREFLEXIA; CLONUS
      PLANTAR REFLEX ABNORMAL
      HEMOGLOBIN OR HEMATOCRIT (LOW)
      PLATELETS (LOW)
      UREA NITROGEN, BLOOD (BUN) (HIGH)
      HEMATURIA

***DIAGNOSES TO BE CONSIDERED***

      THROMBOCYTOPENIC PURPURA, THROMBOTIC        (1)
         R.G.O.F.: 90   R.F.R.: 9 / 9
      PLATELET COUNT; BLOOD SMEAR; BONE MARROW;
      BIOPSY (SKIN, GINGIVA)

      THROMBOCYTOPENIC PURPURA, IDIOPATHIC        (2)
         R.G.O.F.: 80   R.F.R.: 6 / 9
      PLATELET COUNT; BLOOD SMEAR; BONE MARROW

      NEOPLASM OF BLADDER                         (3)
         R.G.O.F.: 80   R.F.R.: 3 / 9
      TRANSURETHRAL BIOPSY

      RENAL FAILURE; UREMIA                       (4)
         R.G.O.F.: 80   R.F.R.: 9 / 9
      SONOGRAM; BIOPSY (KIDNEY)
```

which of the entered findings are considered by Meditel to have an important relationship to each diagnosis.

Knowledge Representation

Meditel represents knowledge of internal medicine diseases by associating clinical findings with disease names. Currently, Meditel represents 1160 disease profiles and 385 clinical findings. For every disease, each finding (and its incidence for that disease) and finding cluster are determined by a literature review as well as by the knowledge and experience of the contributors to and editor of the system. Each finding cluster is also weighted for its importance by the editorial staff. Users of Meditel have the option to identify findings that are prominent or questionable. This information is stored in the computer along with one or more clusters of findings that are suggestive of the disease.

Inference Techniques

Meditel uses a modification of Bayes' theorem, incorporating the incidence and the specificity of the finding in addition to a scoring algorithm to rank the list of possible diagnoses. No details about the scoring algorithm have been published; however, published reports suggest how Meditel ranks diseases. It calculates two entities: the relative goodness of fit (RGOF) and the important finding ratio (IFR). The RGOF is an estimation on a scale of 100 of how well the entered findings fit a given diagnosis relative to the other diagnoses in the system. The RGOF score is calculated using features such as finding specificity and incidence. In addition, the findings are examined by heuristic rules to see if a cluster of findings should evoke a disease. The diagnoses generated by these two processes are given a summary RGOF score and ranked by that score. The IFR is the number of entered findings that Meditel considers to be important for a given diagnosis divided by the total number of entered findings. If, for instance, a disease IFR is 3/10, it means that three of the entered findings can be explained by this disease.

Use of Meditel in Practice

Since Meditel has no facility for browsing the knowledge base, the primary mode of interaction is case analysis. Users enter clinical findings either by typing a three-digit code or by choosing from a hierarchical menu, and they receive a differential diagnosis ranked by RGOF.

An early version of Meditel Adult Diagnostic System was distributed by Elsevier Science Publishing Company, Inc. A new version of the system is expected to be available in 1995.

Quick Medical Reference (QMR)

One of the most widely known and evaluated DDS systems developed for general internal medicine is the INTERNIST-1/Quick Medical Reference program developed at the University of Pittsburgh. Research and development on the INTERNIST-1 project began nearly three decades ago in an attempt to capture the diagnostic expertise of Dr. Jack Myers, a nationally recognized clinician and diagnostician. When presented with findings from a patient's history, physical examination, and laboratory test results, INTERNIST-1 used a heuristic reasoning method with a quasi-probabilistic scoring scheme to suggest likely disease candidates and to guide the physician in the patient's work-up. As it evolved, the system was redesigned to run on personal computers and became the commercial program known as Quick Medical Reference (QMR).

Knowledge Representation

Over 600 disease profiles (Figure 4-4), each consisting of an average of 85 findings, are stored in the knowledge base. There are over 4500 findings in the knowledge base and over 40 000 links described between findings and diseases, diseases and other diseases, or findings and other findings. Each finding in a disease profile has an *evoking strength* and *frequency* weight. Evoking strength is a pseudo-probabilistic categorical measure of the positive predictive value of a finding for a disease. Frequency is a pseudo-probabilistic categorical measure of the sensitivity of a

finding for a disease. Each finding has a disease-independent measure associated with it, known as the *import*, which reflects the clinical significance of the finding or the degree to which it must be explained if present in the patient. In addition to these elements, the knowledge base contains *properties*, which define logical relationships between findings, diseases and findings, or diseases.

Inference Techniques

The diagnostic algorithm used by QMR in case-analysis mode is loosely modeled on the heuristics physicians use to analyze clinical information to arrive at a diagnosis—the hypothetico-deductive approach. An ad hoc score is calculated for each disease hypothesis based on the weight of the evidence in the case. The evoking strength of findings and diseases associated with a given disease add to the score for that disease, while a penalty is assessed against that disease's score, both for findings known

Figure 4-4. The acute appendicitis disease profile from QMR.

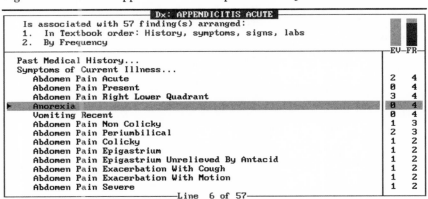

to be absent in the case but expected in the disease and for findings present in the case but unexplained by the disease. The program may generate questions about findings it determines might be useful in sorting out the differential diagnosis.

Use of QMR in Practice

QMR provides a clinician with many functions to access the QMR knowledge base. The developers of QMR classify these functions into three levels. First, a clinician can use QMR as an electronic textbook of medicine to display findings associated with a disease, diseases associated with a finding, or diseases related to a particular disease. Second, a clinician can use QMR as a diagnostic spreadsheet to show how particular groups of diseases and findings may co-occur. In addition, QMR can help the user select the optimal test to rule in or rule out diseases on the differential and can generate simulated cases from the knowledge base for the user to challenge his diagnostic acumen.

Third, a clinician can use QMR as an expert-consultant program to analyze a diagnostic case; in this mode, QMR can provide diagnostic hypotheses containing multiple, pathophysiologically related diseases, or it can critique a diagnostic hypothesis that the clinician suggests.

Table 4-1 lists commercial information for the four DDS programs described in this chapter. A comparison of the programs' features is provided in Table 4-2.

Other Programs Not Evaluated Here

Several other commercially available DDS programs are not discussed in this chapter. The discussion above focuses on systems that cover internal medicine broadly, are generally well known, and whose methods, knowledge content, and evaluation are described in the medical literature. The American College of Physicians' *Software for Internists* contains reviews of several other DDS systems that may be of interest to the reader.

Table 4-1. Diagnostic Decision Support Programs Discussed

Product	Platform	Price*	Publisher or Manufacturer	Address	Phone and Fax Numbers, E-mail Address
DXplain	DOS, Internet	$$ $	Massachusetts General Hospital	Laboratory of Computer Science Massachusetts General Hospital 50 Staniford Street, 5th Floor Boston, MA 02114	Tel: 617-726-3939 Fax: 617-726-8481 E-mail: obarnett@warren.med.harvard.edu
Iliad 4.2	Macintosh, Windows	$$-$$$	Applied Medical Informatics	2681 Parleys Way, Suite 101 Salt Lake City, UT 84109	Tel: 801-464-6200 Fax: 801-464-6201
Meditel Adult Diagnostic System	DOS	$$	Meditel, Inc.	P.O. Box 457 Paoli, PA 19301	N/A
Quick Medical Reference (QMR) 2.03	DOS, Macintosh, Windows	$$	First DataBank	1111 Bayhill Drive Suite 350 San Bruno, CA 94066	Tel: 415-588-5454 800-633-3453 Fax: 415-588-4003

* $ = under $100; $$ = $101 to $500; $$$ = $501 to $1000. Prices are approximate at the time of printing.

Table 4-2. Comparison of Features of Diagnostic Decision Support Programs*

Features		DXplain 4.5	Iliad 4.2	Meditel 2.2	QMR 2.03
Diseases†		2000	930	1160	600
Findings†		4500	11900	385	4500
Links		92 000	?	?	40 000
Inference		Heuristic	Modified Bayes' theorem	Modified Bayes' theorem	Heuristic
Modes:	Case analysis	+	+	+	+
	Critiquing	–	+	–	+
	Disease associations	–	–	–	+
	"Rule in"	–	–	–	+
	"Rule out"	–	–	–	+
	Test costs	–	+	–	–
Help:	Context-specific	–	+	–	+/–
	Online	+	+	–	+
Teaching:	Case simulation	–	+	–	+
Literature citations		+	+	–	+
Therapy:	Treatment suggestions	–	+	–	–

* + means that the program has this feature; – means that the program does not have this feature.
† The comprehensiveness of the knowledge base cannot be determined from these numbers alone.

HOW CAN I SUCCESSFULLY IMPLEMENT DIAGNOSTIC DECISION SUPPORT TECHNOLOGY IN MY PRACTICE?

Methods of Use in Practice

As a group, the DDS programs can be used in three ways: as an electronic knowledge source, as an expert consultant, and as a simulator of clinical cases. We discuss each approach in turn.

AS A KNOWLEDGE SOURCE. Most of the time, clinicians use these programs as an electronic knowledge source. In routine practice, the full DDS function may not be needed often. Typically, the clinician has in mind a fairly direct question, one of those described at the beginning of this chapter: What diseases should I consider given this finding or findings? Is this finding a typical or an atypical feature of a disease I am considering, or can the disease I am considering produce this finding? If the program is available on a computer that is accessible during busy clinic hours, such questions may be addressed in a few minutes or less. These types of questions may be answered using the programs described (except Meditel) without performing a full diagnostic case analysis.

AS A CONSULTANT. If the clinician is confronted with a diagnostically challenging case, he or she may choose to do a full case analysis using one of the DDS programs as an expert consultant. In practice, doing a full case analysis during the patient's visit is difficult, as such an analysis may take 20 to 30 minutes to over an hour, depending on the complexity of the case. Complex cases may have more than 100 positive and negative findings that must be entered by the user. A case entry may be saved, however, so that the same patient information may be re-analyzed on successive visits by adding or deleting only those findings that have changed. Once data for a case has been entered, the most effective way to use a DDS program is to use its knowledge base and functions to iteratively refine a differential diagnosis. For example, the programs may allow a user to check which test is best to rule in or rule out a diagnosis, critique a diagnostic hypothesis under consideration, view the conditions associated with a disease hypothesis, or view the selected literature citations. In this manner, the user is interacting with the program's knowledge base, using the program's functions to refine her or his diagnostic hypotheses.

AS A SIMULATOR. Some of these programs (Iliad and QMR) can be used to simulate cases. The program can randomly (or from a user-defined focus area) select a disease from its knowledge base and create a simulated patient with that disease. The user then asks the computer whether the patient has particular findings. At any time, the user can assert his diagnosis and compare it with the computer-generated diagnosis. The simulation feature is an enjoyable way to refresh your knowledge of particular diagnoses and is also useful in teaching medical students differential diagnosis.

Diagnostic Accuracy

Whether one of these programs is being used only as an electronic knowledge source or in the full diagnostic decision support mode, the user should understand the limitations of the program's knowledge base to properly interpret the output generated by the program. None of the programs described has every disease in internal medicine—not to mention the entire universe of possible diseases from all specialties together—programmed in its knowledge base. The program cannot inform the user that the most plausible disease hypothesis may not be in the knowledge base—it simply attempts to make a diagnosis from among those diseases programmed into the knowledge base to fit the findings input by the user. In this situation, a set of findings may cause the user to think of a certain disease or problem area that is not in the knowledge base. The differential diagnosis generated by the program may look ridiculous if an obvious diagnostic consideration is not presented because it is not in the knowledge base. Similarly, none of the knowledge bases described contain all possible findings. Thus, the user may have a clear finding concept in mind that cannot be found in the knowledge base and cannot be put into the program for analysis. This limitation is much more obvious to the user and forces either an attempt to conceive how the program developers might have stated the finding concept in their own terms or to accept that the program does not have the finding concept in its knowledge base. In this situation, the user may decide not to pursue further analysis with the program because important findings for that case are not represented in the knowledge base.

Currency of the knowledge base is also important because new diagnostic tests are continually emerging. The user must always keep in mind potential delays between availability of new information and its incorporation into the knowledge base.

These limitations in the program's knowledge base and the user's facility in translating an observed clinical finding concept into the language and semantics of the program obviously affect the accuracy and utility of the knowledge derived from the program. Fortunately, an experienced clinician usually knows when the DDS program is "making sense" or not.

In addition to the limitations described above, the user must also understand conceptually the way in which the programs make associations or inference. Although each program provides useful information to clinicians, each one also uses a different approach with varying strengths and weaknesses.

The Bayesian approach, which underlies Iliad and Meditel, relies on estimates of disease prevalence and conditional probabilities to characterize the strength of the relation between findings and disease. If any of these numbers are biased, the program may misinterpret evidence and give a misleading differential. For example, the prevalence of pulmonary tuberculosis (TB) is higher in New York City than in Denver. Thus, if a program used the New York value for the prior probability of TB, a user in Denver might see an overstated probability of TB. Similarly, bias in the numbers used to characterize the strength of the relations between findings and disease may also lead to spurious results. Ideally, the prior and conditional probabilities of a Bayesian expert diagnostic system should reflect the local experience where the program is being used. Other problems may arise using Bayesian approaches, but they are beyond the scope of this chapter.

With associational or heuristic reasoning techniques such as those used by QMR and DXplain, problems similar to those described above may arise and be more difficult to detect. Like Bayesian approaches, associational reasoning may also fail to properly adjust the prior probability of disease. Such systems may have difficulty both in diagnosing more than one disease and in focusing on relevant hypotheses, depending on the richness of the rule base. Both Bayesian and associational techniques typically are unable to make use of "deep" models of pathophysiology, anatomy, or time that are indispensable for the human diagnostician. Thus, while these tools may provide an encyclopedic knowledge base, they are only a cognitive aid to human diagnostic reasoning and never a substitute.

Access to the DDS System

As discussed in the Introduction to this book, clinical information management software is more likely to be used when the computer is near the work flow in the office (or elsewhere) and has enough functionality to be generally useful to the practitioner. That is, if the computer has only a DDS application and no other, the user may be less inclined to turn to the computer for diagnostic assistance. But if the computer is already being used for other clinical information management tasks such as access to CD-ROM reference discs, MEDLINE access, or other clinically oriented applications, the user is more likely to also use the DDS application.

At least four strategies can be considered for accessing DDS systems and other clinical tools: 1) Locate the computer in the physician's work room (or office), 2) in the examination room, 3) or at home or in another setting apart from the clinical environment, or 4) load the software on a portable computer. Many users discover uses for these tools in more than one setting. Pick the approach that works best for you.

Selecting a DDS Program

Selecting one of the DDS tools we have described can be done much like selecting any other software application. Users are interested in the programs available on the computer platform they have—all four DDS programs are available for IBM-compatibles; only Iliad and QMR are currently available for Macintosh computers. Many users are influenced by other users who already have one of the programs and who can give a detailed account of its strengths and weaknesses. Finding a current user and asking direct questions is probably the

best way to decide which program is right for you. The Introduction to this book offers sound strategies for choosing among available software products (*see* Introduction, Making the Best of What Is Available). The authors also offer a computer-aided diagnosis workshop at the American College of Physicians' Annual Session, which may be useful for its overview of current systems and hands-on trial of each system.

Training and Education

To become an effective and knowledgeable user of one of these DDS tools, you must familiarize yourself both with the basic features and functionality of the program and with the limitations of the knowledge base and inference techniques described above. These complex tools have been created to support, but not replace, a complex process—diagnostic reasoning—and they have strengths and weaknesses that must be appreciated by the user to properly interpret and use the information provided by the program.

Each of the programs can be set up in less than 30 minutes on a computer and used immediately by the computer-literate user. Review of the manual and tutorial, however, is strongly recommended to understand fully the capabilities of these powerful programs. New users should "play" with the program to explore its knowledge base and functionality. Such users may want to pick one or two interesting and useful functions, learn them well, and practice them often. The electronic textbook functions tend to have a higher benefit-to-cost ratio for beginners. As you become familiar with the program, adding new functions to your repertoire is easier.

The user should practice identifying questions that may be addressed with these tools and determining how they are used to answer specific questions. Over time, the user will come to understand how the program designers built the knowledge base and to appreciate the differences in how the user might state a clinical finding or disease versus how the program designers state the same concept in the knowledge base. Time invested in learning to understand and use these tools properly increases their utility in practice.

In the Future

Increasingly, physicians may be expected to use DDS tools and their descendants as they become integral components of our clinical information management environment or the computer-based patient record. Diagnostic decision support tools will be complemented by and integrated with therapeutic decision support tools (see Chapter 5) and information retrieval tools (see Chapter 9) to provide the physician with a comprehensive clinical information management environment to help provide the best care possible for his or her patients.

5

THERAPEUTIC DECISION SUPPORT

Paul N. Gorman, MD, FACP; and Barry H. Blumenfeld, MD, MS

This chapter covers software products designed to help clinicians select and dispense therapy. We have included information about software for a range of tasks, including choosing drug treatments, obtaining information about medications, checking for drug interactions, writing and renewing prescriptions, tracking patient medication regimens, and providing information about medications to the patient. Also covered are products for diet therapy, including diet analysis and meal-planning software.

HOW CAN THERAPEUTIC DECISION SUPPORT SOFTWARE HELP ME IN MY PRACTICE?

Having questions about treatment is one of the commonest reasons for practicing physicians to seek information, and often they must consult several sources to find what they need. Complex multidrug regimens increase the likelihood of adverse drug reactions and interactions; complications from such regimens are reported to cause a significant proportion of hospital admissions. Changes in health care organization are increasing the time constraints on practitioners, making it all the more difficult to find the time to obtain additional information when it is needed. For these reasons, practitioners can benefit from software that provides rapid access to accurate, up-to-date information about drug therapy and that assists in the process of selecting, dispensing, tracking, and renewing medications.

Benefits

The benefits of computer-based therapeutic decision support (TDS) are of four main types: 1) the electronic format of the information; 2) the integration of information tools into the practitioner's work flow; 3) automation (for example, reminders); and 4) the enhanced capability for quality control.

ELECTRONIC FORMAT. Electronic information sources offer major advantages over printed text. Their compact size means that vast amounts of information can be stored in a small physical space, even on hand-held devices such as "palmtop" computers. Information in digital form can be updated and edited more readily than printed information and allows for much more extensive indexing than a table of contents or printed index, which leads to flexible, powerful, and extremely rapid search and retrieval of information.

INTEGRATION OF TOOLS. Integration of computer-based TDS tools into the flow of daily practice makes the information available during the patient care process when it is most needed and can be used most readily. Integration of drug information sources with other medical knowledge sources such as electronic textbooks allows users to search for information about a disease and its treatment using a single clinical computing tool. Integration of prescription-writing software with drug interaction software and patient-specific data allows for automatic screening for adverse drug interactions and patient allergies as prescriptions are entered, before printing or dispensing. This important function is cumbersome with print-based resources (especially with multidrug regimens) and is often neglected. Integration with patient education software allows information about medications to be printed (and documented) at the time of prescription. Integration with an electronic medical record facilitates later retrieval of patient medication lists for prescription review and renewal and can form the basis for practitioners to examine treatment outcomes.

AUTOMATION. Automation of certain processes of care can help practitioners to overcome the limits of human memory and the constraints of time. Automatic screening for allergies and drug interactions at the time of prescription entry has already been mentioned. Automatic reminder systems can be used to prompt physicians to obtain appropriate monitoring of drug side effects and blood levels at the time of prescription renewal or to recall patients for scheduled follow-up, such as for serial immunizations.

QUALITY CONTROL. Whatever your practice situation, quality control is an issue. While physicians have always been concerned with quality, their efforts are increasingly subjected to outside scrutiny. In many cases, the words "quality control" are heard with dread or outright loathing when they are associated with cost controls and managed care. But like it or not, physicians are now coming under the cold gaze of efficiency planners, whose ideas have forever changed modern industry. In the competitive atmosphere of medicine today, patient satisfaction counts, and using TDS software is sometimes a way to increase patient satisfaction. It also leads to better documentation in most cases and, if used consistently, can cut down on the frequency of adverse drug effects.

Using such software will, at least at first, invariably eat up more of your precious time—no matter what the advertisements tell you about the ease of implementation. But the bottom line is that physicians care deeply about the quality and results of the care they provide, and therapeutic support software offers practitioners a new and powerful means of examining and improving that care.

Limitations

The actual and potential disadvantages of TDS software must also be considered. First is cost, including the initial cost of the software, annual upgrade or relicensing charges, and the cost of any necessary additional hardware such as computer memory, storage, or CD-ROM equipment. Also included in total cost is the training of the physicians and staff who will use the product. Second are problems with usability—the decreased efficiency in reading from a computer screen compared with reading from paper, differences in interface design that require a separate learning process for each product used, and the constraints and changes in office work flow that may result from incorporating the product into your practice. Third is the software itself. Each product is only as good as the knowledge base (information source) it uses, and this information may be inadequate or may become outdated unless properly maintained. Further, the search software may not be optimized to help the user retrieve relevant information from the database.

Finally, there is the potential danger of placing too much faith in information because it comes from the computer. Although human memory is imperfect and can benefit from the assistance of clinical computing tools, no substitute exists for the good judgment of thoughtful clinicians in making treatment decisions.

WHAT THERAPEUTIC DECISION SUPPORT PRODUCTS ARE AVAILABLE?

In this section, we discuss the major categories of TDS software and representative products in each category. We do not provide an exhaustive product listing or software review. To learn details about specific products discussed and others not mentioned, consult other sources such as product vendors and the American College of Physicians' compendium *Software for Internists*. The strategies given in the Introduction to this book should also help you identify and evaluate TDS software, and, in addition, the Appendix lists other useful resources. Note that software primarily meant for other tasks but which may also be used for TDS (for example, MEDLINE searching to obtain information about treatment) is covered elsewhere in this book. Also not covered in this chapter are products meant for tasks not usually done by physicians, such as pharmacokinetics and pharmacy management. A list of the products discussed in this section is given in Table 5-1.

Therapeutic decision support products can be classified according to the task they are designed to assist. We will look at the following categories:

- Choosing a treatment
- Obtaining basic drug information (for example, indications, adverse reactions, and dosing)
- Checking for drug interactions

Table 5-1. Therapeutic Decision Support Products Discussed

Product	Platform	Price*	Publisher or Manufacturer	Address	Phone and Fax Numbers
AskRx Plus	Windows	$$	First DataBank	1111 Bayhill Drive, Suite 350 San Bruno, CA 94066	Tel: 415-588-5454 Fax: 415-588-4003
Computerized Health Diet	DOS	$$	INPS	P.O. Box 7847 Overland Park, KS 66207	Tel: 800-798-6419 Fax: 913-648-8316
EASY DOC Script	DOS	$$	EASY DOC Corp.	P.O. Box 1474 Wilson, NC 27894	Tel: 919-243-7246 Fax: 919-243-7247
Electronic Drug Reference 4.5	DOS	$$ single user	Clinical Reference Systems, Ltd.	7100 East Belleview Avenue Suite 208 Greenwood Village, CO 80111	Tel: 800-237-8401 303-220-1661 Fax: 303-220-1685
Immunization Manager	DOS, Windows	$$	Medical Software Products	591 West Hamilton Avenue Suite 205 Campbell, CA 95008	Tel: 800-444-4570 Fax: 408-370-3393
The Medical Letter Drug Interactions	DOS, Macintosh, Windows	$$	The Medical Letter, Inc.	1000 Main Street New Rochelle, NY 10801-7537	Tel: 914-235-0500 Fax: 914-632-1733
Medication Advisor	DOS	$$	Clinical Reference Systems, Ltd.	7100 East Belleview Avenue Suite 208 Greenwood Village, CO 80111	Tel: 800-237-8401 303-220-1661 Fax: 303-220-1685
Nutri-Calc Plus	Macintosh	$$	CAMDE Corp.	449 East Saratoga Street Gilbert, AZ 85296	Tel: 602-926-2632 Fax: 602-926-2632
Patient Drug Education-PC	DOS	$$	Drug Facts and Comparisons	111 West Port Plaza, Suite 400 St. Louis, MO 63146-0554	Tel: 314-878-2515 Fax: 314-878-5563

* $ = under $100; $$ = $101 to $500; $$$ = $501 to $1000. Prices are approximate at the time of printing.

- Writing and printing prescriptions and tracking patient medication regimens
- Providing patient education about the therapy
- Analyzing and planning diet therapy.

Examples of products that perform these tasks are provided in Table 5-2. (Note that one of the authors of this chapter [BB] is affiliated with First DataBank, which publishes AskRx and AskAdvice.)

Choosing Treatments

Special-purpose programs are available to support decisions about treatment of specific conditions. These products include Travel Care (health advice for travelers); TP Write (for preparing mental health treatment plans); and Immunization Manager (for planning and reminding about immunization schedules). Each offers the advantage of patient-specific,

Table 5-1. (*Continued*)

Product	Platform	Price*	Publisher or Manufacturer	Address	Phone and Fax Numbers
PDR Drug Interactions, Side Effects, and Indications	DOS	$$-$$$	Medical Economics Data	5 Paragon Drive Montvale, NJ 07645	Tel: 800-232-7379 Fax: 201-573-4956
PDR Library on CD-ROM	DOS	$$$	Medical Economics Data	5 Paragon Drive Montvale, NJ 07645	Tel: 800-232-7379 Fax: 201-573-4956
Pharmaceuticals 3.0	DOS	$$	Edu-Calc	27953 Cabot Road Laguna Niguel, CA 92677	Tel: 800-677-7001 Fax: 714-582-1445
PharmacoLogic	DOS	$$$	MedicaLogic	15400 N.W. Greenbrier Parkway Suite 400 Beaverton, OR 97006	Tel: 503-531-7000 Fax: 503-531-7001
Script Consultant-DM	DOS	$$	Rapha Group Software, Inc.	433 Carson Road St. Louis, MO 63135	Tel: 314-521-0808
S-O-A-P Drug Interaction and Prescription Writer Program	DOS	$$	Patient Medical Records, Inc.	901 Tahoka Road Brownfield, TX 79316	Tel: 800-285-7627 Fax: 806-637-4283
SuperDOC! Prescription Writer	DOS	$$	SuperDOC! Software	P.O. Box 1113 Harrisonburg, VA 22801	Tel: 800-541-0322 Fax: 703-433-7731
TP Write	DOS	$$	Reason House Software	101 East Chesapeake Avenue Towson, MD 21286	Tel: 410-321-7270 Fax: 410-823-6204
Travel Care 2.0	Macintosh, Windows	$$	Care Ware, Inc.	9559 Poole Street La Jolla, CA 92037	Tel: 619-455-1484 Fax: 619-455-5429

disease-specific treatment planning. However, each is a stand-alone product, requiring separate entry and maintenance of patient data, without allowing integration with an existing patient information system or other TDS products. Users interact with these programs by entering relevant information about the patient. A knowledge base within the program then generates patient-specific treatment recommendations. Reviews of this type of special-purpose prod-

uct generally indicate that they perform their intended functions well but that the lack of ability to integrate with clinical systems is a major drawback.

General clinical references are also useful resources when deciding whether to treat and with what agent. For general medicine, electronic textbooks such as SAM-CD (*see* Chapter 9) and the electronic Washington University Manual of Medical Therapeutics (Franklin palmtop version; *see* Chapter 10) may

Table 5-2. Therapeutic Decision Support Programs and Their Functions*

Product	Function							
	Assists Treatment Choice	Provides Basic Drug Information	Checks for Drug Interactions	Writes Prescriptions	Tracks Medication Regimens	Provides Patient Education Handouts	Provides Meal Planning	Provides Diet Analysis
AskRx Plus	+	+	+	+	+	+	–	–
Computerized Health Diet	–	–	–	–	–	–	+	–
Easy DOC Script	–	–	–	+	+	–	–	–
Electronic Drug Reference 4.5	–	Partial	–	–	–	+	–	–
Immunization Manager	+	–	–	–	+	–	–	–
Medication Advisor	–	–	–	–	–	+	–	–
Nutri-Calc Plus	–	–	–	–	–	–	–	+
Patient Drug Education-PC	–	–	–	–	–	+	–	–
PDR Drug Interactions	–	–	+	–	–	–	–	–

* + means that the program has this function; – means that the program does not have this function.

provide convenient access to information needed for therapeutic decision making. Treatment information is also included in some diagnostic decision support software such as Iliad 4.2 (*see* Chapter 4).

Two types of information that are increasingly available in electronic format—practice guidelines and trial registries—deserve mention here because of their potential usefulness for selecting effective therapies. Up-to-date versions of published practice guidelines and practice parameters are now available electronically from various organizations,

including the Agency for Health Care Policy and Research (practice guidelines); National Institutes of Health (Consensus Development Conference reports); and the Physicians' Data Query (PDQ) cancer information database (accessible through the NIH Internet gopher and various CD-ROM products). The American College of Physicians' *Clinical Practice Guidelines* will also be available electronically in 1995.

Online registries such as the Oxford Database of Perinatal Trials from the Cochrane Collaborations

Table 5-2. (*Continued*)

Product	Function							
	Assists Treatment Choice	Provides Basic Drug Information	Checks for Drug Interactions	Writes Prescriptions	Tracks Medication Regimens	Provides Patient Education Handouts	Provides Meal Planning	Provides Diet Analysis
PDR Library on CD-ROM	−	+	+	−	−	−	−	−
Pharmaceuticals 3.0	−	Partial	−	−	−	−	−	−
PharmacoLogic	−	−	+	+	+	+	−	−
Pocket PDR	−	Partial	−	−	−	−	−	−
S-O-A-P Drug Interaction Program	−	−	+	−	+	+	−	−
Script Consultant	−	−	+	+	+	+	−	−
STAT!-Ref CD-ROM	+	+	+	−	−	−	−	−
SuperDOC! Prescription Writer	−	−	−	+	+	−	−	−
The Medical Letter Drug Interactions	−	−	+	−	−	−	−	−
TP Write	+	−	−	−	+	−	−	−
Travel Care 2.0	+	−	−	−	−	+	−	−

provide electronic access to systematic overviews of randomized trials of therapy. These registries are constantly updated as new trials are published so that results are available electronically well before the reviews could be published in printed form. They differ from bibliographic databases such as MEDLINE in that they contain only information from randomized controlled trials, where the trials have been expertly appraised for validity and the information has been organized into summary form. In the future, as the content of online registries developed by international efforts such as the Cochrane Collaborations expands to include more and more conditions and treatments, practitioners will be able to use them to access the latest, best evidence about the effects of treatments.

Obtaining Basic Drug Information

Full-text information about pharmaceuticals is available in a number of stand-alone and integrated computer-based products. Most are based on existing printed sources of drug information such as those of the American Society of Hospital Pharmacists (ASHP), the *USP Dictionary of Drug Names,* or the *Physicians' Desk Reference (PDR).* As with their paper counterparts, the information provided about each drug in these computerized versions generally includes categories such as adverse effects, interactions, and contraindications. Usually the software interface provides tools for accessing and displaying this information more rapidly than with the paper version. The knowledge bases for these products differ in content and purpose, so products should be selected with this fact in mind. Issues to consider include completeness of the database (are all relevant drugs such as prescription and nonprescription drugs included?); comprehensiveness of the information about each drug (are all relevant categories of information included?); and organization (is the information organized optimally for use by physicians?).

Desktop software for retrieving the full text of drug information include CD-ROM–based products that contain a single comprehensive drug information source such as PDR on CD-ROM (Figure 5-1) or multiple information sources such as STAT!-Ref CD-ROM (*see* Chapter 9), which contains multiple texts that are separately licensed, including AMA Drug Evaluations, USP Drug Information, American Hospital Formulary Service Drug Information, and The Medical Letter Handbook of Drug Interactions, among others. Non–CD-ROM products, whose information may be stored on your computer's hard disk, generally contain a smaller information base by including either fewer drugs or less information

about each drug. Examples include Pharmaceuticals 3.0 and Electronic Drug Reference 4.5.

Portable products such as the Pocket PDR module for the Franklin Digital Book system (*see* Chapter 10)

Figure 5-1. PDR Library on CD-ROM. Top. Screen shows the main menu of PDR Library. **Bottom.** Screen shows a drug description, partly obscured by the menu of subtopics of drug information.

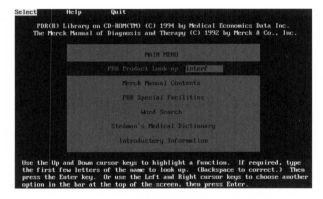

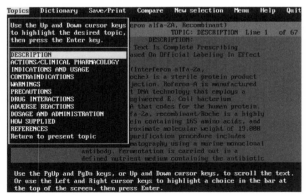

are compact and therefore readily accessible (if you can remember where you left them). The database in these products is usually limited to only the most often-used information such as indications, adverse reactions, and dosage and administration; their compact size is both an advantage and a disadvantage since the small screen size limits the amount of information displayed.

The model for using basic drug-information software is roughly similar to that of traditional, printed texts. Either you start with the table of contents and choose a topic of interest, or you use the electronic index to locate items of interest. One advantage of software over paper is the capability to search for multiple terms at the same time and to search the entire text for all occurrences of those terms. In most cases, the information can be viewed in outline form, allowing you to quickly scan or skip to the needed information. With many desktop systems, the text may be printed for later review. These drug-information programs contain a fixed database and do not require any data entry. Most products offer or include periodic updates of new medications and prescribing information.

Checking for Drug Interactions

Software that enables the practitioner to check for adverse drug interactions is available in stand-alone and integrated products. Stand-alone products for desktop computers, such as The Medical Letter Drug Interactions Software, allow entry of a patient medication profile, which is searched for interactions among all of the drugs. The program then displays a list of each pair of drugs with a reported interaction, the nature of the interaction, any recommended substitutions or other actions, and references to the literature reporting the interaction. The Franklin Handbook of Drug Interactions offers a similar capability on a hand-held palmtop computer (*see* Chapter 10). Important differentiating features among drug interaction programs include the scope and currency of their knowledge bases, the extent to which identified interactions are referenced, the ease with which drug names are entered, and their connectivity with other clinical information systems. Integrated products that combine drug interaction screening with other functions are further noted in the section Integrated Products.

Writing Prescriptions and Tracking Patient Medications

Basic prescription-writing software products such as EASY DOC Script and SuperDOC! Prescription Writer allow the practitioner to enter and print multiple prescriptions for a given patient; these programs also maintain an electronic patient medication profile to facilitate medication tracking and prescription renewals.

To use a basic prescription-writing program, you enter the name of a medication and then select from a list of preparations of that medication found in the program's database. Once the preparation is selected, the software allows you to enter the dose, route, *Sig.* (instructions for patient use of medication), and number of refills. Some more sophisticated programs enter default values that reflect typical prescriptions for each drug; the user can then edit each value as needed. Many programs provide other tools to minimize typing and speed prescription entry. For example, there may be pick-lists for choosing common dosing intervals and medication routes and various index navigation aids that permit medication selection with just a few mouse clicks or keystrokes.

The prescription-writing programs store information about your practice, for example, your name, address, Drug Enforcement Agency (DEA) number, and medical license number. Once all the key information is complete, the prescription can easily be stored and printed. With the printing, however, some logistic issues do come into play. For example, special paper may be required for the small size of prescriptions. Using such paper requires either a dedicated printer or switching between standard and prescription-sized paper. In either case, the printer must be able to accommodate the prescription paper.

At the heart of these programs lies some sort of database that enables you to build medication profiles for each patient. Each profile allows you to reap the benefits of the initial work of entering the prescriptions. Refills of prescriptions can usually be easily generated after recalling the profile. Similarly, prescriptions can be modified and new medications can be added with less effort than that required to create the profile initially. Whether or not the profile has changed, legible, current medication lists can be printed for the patient or the medical record, or both.

The database features of prescription management software may be invaluable for auditing your prescribing patterns. They may also literally be lifesavers when a drug is recalled or strong warnings are added

owing to severe adverse effects. Physicians who use this software may be able to identify in minutes all the patients for whom such a drug or combination of drugs has been prescribed. This type of information can be extremely time consuming, expensive, and difficult (if not impossible) to obtain for a frequently used drug in a large, busy practice.

Providing Patient Education

Several of the software products already described can produce educational materials for patients in addition to their other functions. Stand-alone products for this purpose include Patient Drug Education-PC and Medication Advisor. AskAdvice, based on the volume *USP DI Advice for the Patient,* can be used as a stand-alone product or in combination with its companion product, AskRx Plus (*see* Chapter 6). Some products allow only minimal editing or customization, such as printing the physician or practice name in a header at the top of the page, while others allow more customization of the instructions given to the patient. To use this kind of software, like the products mentioned above, you enter all or part of the name of the medication of interest, prompting the program to search its database and present a list of preparations that match your search entry. You then select the desired medication from the list and print the patient instructions.

Integrated Products

Integrated TDS software allows the practitioner to perform several functions with a single product. Using

AskRx Plus, for example, a practitioner can retrieve basic drug information, check for adverse drug interactions, write and renew prescriptions, and maintain and print individual patient medication lists (Figure 5-2). For each patient, a patient profile can be entered, including a problem list, medications, allergies, and the like. Then, at each patient encounter, you enter the patient's name to review the patient's problem list and active medications. You can search by disease to identify treatments used for a specific disorder, or you can search for a specific drug. If you add the medication to the patient's medication list, the program automatically checks for any interactions with the patient's other medications and notifies you if any are found. You can then print prescriptions for any medication on the list without having to rewrite the prescribing information by hand. The companion product,

AskAdvice, enables you to easily print patient instructions as well. The AskRX Plus software maintains a partial patient profile but does not function as a complete electronic medical record. PharmacoLogic software, when integrated with the same vendor's ClinicaLogic module (*see* Chapter 2), works similarly but integrates prescription writing and automatic checking for drug interactions with a full electronic medical record system; this program, however, does not offer access to full-text drug information.

Other products that provide multiple TDS functions include Script Consultant and S-O-A-P Drug Interaction and Prescription Writer Program. These programs combine prescription writing and medication tracking with drug-interaction screening and printing of patient education material.

Prescribing Diet Therapy

Nutrition is increasingly recognized as a critical component of health care. Nutrition-related software can help physicians manage within their practice this aspect of therapy, which is often referred to dietitians or handled in a superficial manner. Two types of software are available for diet therapy: meal planning and diet analysis. Meal-planning products such as Computerized Health Diet allow the clinician to enter individual nutrient restrictions for each patient and then combine this patient profile with current dietary guidelines to create an individualized meal plan. This tool is useful in managing patients who require low-fat, low-sodium, or other frequently recommended diets. Diet analysis programs such as Nutri-Calc Plus require the user to enter a list of foods consumed by the patient and then

Figure 5-2. AskRx Plus. Screen shows a patient's demographic information and medication list.

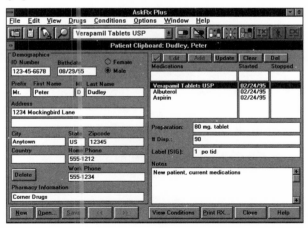

analyze the nutrient content of the diet and allow the user to display and print the results of the analysis.

HOW CAN I SUCCESSFULLY IMPLEMENT THERAPEUTIC DECISION SUPPORT TECHNOLOGY IN MY PRACTICE?

Incorporating TDS software into your practice can be as straightforward as installing the product and starting to search for information, or it can be more complex, involving an alteration in practice routines to accommodate electronic prescription management. The ways in which these products are used by physicians are as varied as the personalities of the physicians themselves. However, some generalizations can be made. In most cases, the software is being used on a stand-alone basis; that is, it is installed on a single computer in the office and is neither networked nor integrated with other office software. While this situation is unfortunate, it is understandable, since few of the packages support integration and most are not available in network versions. Many physicians have started using notebook computers for these clinical applications so that they can take the software with them on rounds or when traveling (*see* Chapter 10). Some physicians are regularly using drug information and interaction software packages on hand-held computers like the Hewlett Packard 200 LX Palmtop PC (*see* Chapter 10).

Implementation Imperatives

Many physicians have successfully incorporated TDS software into their practices and will attest to its benefit. By carefully evaluating your functional requirements and setting, you can expect to do so as well. To make the implementation process successful, certain rules of thumb are worth following:

- Evaluate your practice environment
- Know what you want
- Find out what you already have
- Assess your tolerance for technology
- Do your homework
- Test the software yourself
- Plan for installation and training
- Anticipate updates and maintenance.

Evaluate Your Practice Environment

Begin by asking a lot of questions. Where do you spend most of your time? Are you office or hospital based? If you are office based, how often are you someplace other than the office? How long do you typically allow for seeing a patient? Are you primary care oriented, or are you a specialist? How sick are your patients, and do you tend to see primarily one age group? Answers to these questions may have an effect on the types of software you will find most useful.

For instance, if you are primarily hospital based and do not spend most of your time near a single desktop, you may want to consider drug information and interaction software that easily fits on a notebook computer. On the other hand, if you are primary care oriented and spend a great deal of time counseling and writing prescriptions for a large, stable geriatric population in a single location, for example, then you might benefit significantly from implementing several integrated therapeutic information products such as software for drug information, writing and tracking prescriptions, detecting drug interactions, generating patient drug handouts, and prescribing diet therapy. Although a stand-alone product that integrates these functions would likely be useful in this setting, one that integrates fully with a practice management system might be even more desirable.

Know What You Want

Your expectations are more likely to be met if they are clearly stated. First, identify and list in order of priority those functions you expect the software to perform. Will you be satisfied with a stand-alone system for drug interactions or diet prescriptions, or will you require an integrated therapy management system? Next, begin thinking about the types of software that will best satisfy your functional requirements and preferences. Finally, consider the implications that your requirements will have on the necessary computer hardware to run that software. Software that runs on your existing hardware but does not meet your needs is no bargain.

Find Out What You Already Have

What systems or functions are already in place in your practice setting? Are you already using clinical software? If so, how will you begin to integrate packages? Entering data redundantly quickly becomes tedious. When evaluating a software package, always ask about its information importing and exporting capacities as well as whether it can communicate with other programs in real time. Also look at the equipment you currently own. Is it compatible with the software you are evaluating? Will you have to buy expensive new equipment? Were you planning to upgrade your current equipment soon anyway?

For some hospital and HMO-based physicians, all prescriptions are processed through a single pharmacy system which maintains patient medication profiles and checks for drug interactions, so there is no need to duplicate these functions. For some office-based physicians, the office medical record system already in place may offer integrated pharmaceutical information or drug interaction modules as optional features. If you are not using such a system, you may want to explore upgrading to one.

Assess Your Tolerance for Technology

Do you prefer a turnkey system, which requires no installation or modification efforts on your part and has minimal room for customization? Or would you rather have a more flexible product that allows for some customization to meet your specific needs but requires more time and effort by you and your staff? Are you willing to enter patient data in order to use the product, or do you simply want to look up drug information and keep your current patient data (medical record) system unchanged? Entering prescriptions for all your patients carries a high up-front cost but can repay you handsomely when generating refills, dealing with a product recall, or automatically checking for interactions. Remember to make sure that you can export this hard-earned data in case you want to change prescription management systems.

Do Your Homework

Do not rely solely on product information from the vendor. For the products that interest you, look for reviews in publications such as *Software for Internists* from the American College of Physicians, *Medical Software Reviews, MD Computing,* the book review section of many journals, and occasionally computer trade magazines. Contact current users of the software to ask whether it performs as expected and what problems have occurred.

Test the Software Yourself

Make sure the software you select performs the functions you have in mind. Ask the vendor for a working demonstration version, or order the product at a time when you can adequately test it in your practice setting during a money-back guarantee period. For large complex systems, contact current users of the system and, if possible, visit their site to see them using the software in practice. Remember to consider issues such as portability, usability, primary input devices (typing versus a mouse), network compatibility, memory requirements, and adequacy of the knowledge base.

Plan for Installation and Training

Even fairly straightforward products have a learning curve and can at first require some adjustments to your usual pace and work flow as you learn how best to incorporate them into your practice. Sophisticated, integrated software products such as those that combine therapeutic decision support with an electronic medical record may save time and expense in the long run; initially, though, planning and patience are required to bring all practitioners and office staff up to speed with the product and to take advantage of its functions. You should prepare to invest time and effort, for example, in initially creating patient medication profiles. There may be a need for additional technical support, dedicated training time, and a project "evangelist" to carry the process through. Some companies offer training for a fee or refer you to a local "expert" user who has volunteered to help new users. Most software companies offer free telephone support, but you should check to make sure.

Anticipate Updates and Maintenance

One advantage of TDS software is the up-to-date information it can provide. This feature also means periodic updates or relicensing of the software to keep the information current and take advantage of improvements. You should inquire about the updating costs, contents, and mechanisms. You should think twice about using knowledge-based products that do not provide for regular updates since therapeutic information evolves continually. You should also check whether you can return the software if you are not satisfied after a trial period—usually 30 days.

Therapeutic Decision Support: One Working Scenario

The clinicians at Anytown Adult Medicine, PC, had on many occasions informally discussed their frustrations with writing and rewriting prescriptions, and they finally decided to do something about it. Following one gripe session, the discussion turned to computers. Several members of the group were using home computers for various personal uses and had heard about computer software for selecting and dispensing medications. The group agreed to explore their options for putting such tools to use in their practice.

They began by creating a "wish list" of functions they hoped the software would perform. Each member of the group championed a different area of concern:

- Sam Smith, MD, a geriatrician, felt that avoiding drug-drug interactions in patients on complicated, multiple-drug regimens was a constant challenge.

- Mary Miles, MD, a general internist, was concerned about prescriptions written in the group's after-hours urgent-care clinic, when access to information about the patient's other medical problems and medications was limited.

- Bill Martin, MD, the senior physician in the group, and Carol Jones, MD, the group's newest member, both objected to the inefficiency of repeatedly recording the same medication information in multiple places—in a progress note for their own records, on a prescription form for the pharmacist, on a medication-instruction sheet for the patient, and sometimes on a separate approval form for the patient's managed-care organization.

- Tom Turner, NP, a nurse-practitioner who had recently joined the group, was looking for a comprehensive, up-to-date source of information about pharmaceuticals.

With their wish list complete, they divided up the task of finding computer software to meet their needs. Bill, who had been with the group longest, offered to review the information about their practice management and billing package to learn whether additional functions were available and whether the software could be integrated with other products. Tom, whose children used a multimedia electronic encyclopedia on their CD-ROM–equipped home computer, agreed to find out about computer-based drug information sources. Mary and Carol volunteered to look into software for printing prescriptions and patient handouts. Sam had already obtained demonstration versions of some drug interaction software and agreed to show these to the group at a future meeting.

Members of the group prepared a list of existing software, looked in books and medical magazines for product reviews, and obtained demonstration or trial versions of the software, where available. It turned out that their office billing and practice management package, purchased a decade earlier, offered no additional functions and had no ability to be integrated with other computer software. Therefore, if they were going to track patient information, demographic data would have to be entered separately for each system. Many other functions on their wish list were available in existing software packages, either separately or in combination, but no one product appeared to meet all of their present needs.

After examining the information they had collected, the group decided on a two-stage plan. In the long term, they expected to eventually replace their office management and billing package. As they approached that decision, they would keep in mind the need for expanded capabilities in their office system, such as therapeutic decision support and an electronic medical record. In the near term, they would evaluate several stand-alone products that offered many of the functions they desired, paying special attention to the time and effort needed to learn to use each product and to how it could fit into their office work flow. They would choose one of these products for the group to use over the next few years.

Each clinician at Anytown Adult Medicine now has a new computer workstation in his or her workspace, and each workstation is connected to an office network so that group members can share access to the same information about their patients. Working in the after-hours clinic, Tom Turner, NP, sees a patient of Dr. Smith's, an elderly woman with acute bronchitis. Using their new TDS system, Tom first obtains a list of antibiotics used for treatment of bronchitis in adults and reads about the indications, dosing, and adverse effects of each. Because basic clinical information about most patients has been entered into the new system as these patients have been seen, Tom can access a list of this patient's medical problems and medications. He takes a few moments to add "acute bronchitis" to her problem list, and then adds the antibiotic he has chosen to her medication list. The system automatically checks for interactions between the antibiotic and her other medications and verifies that none are listed. Next, Tom uses the system to print a prescription for the antibiotic and a handout for the patient with information about the new medication, documenting all this in the process. When the patient incidentally requests refills for several of her other medications, he reviews her medication list to verify the medications, doses, and dates of the last refills and then prints the prescriptions.

The practitioners at Anytown Adult Medicine have successfully incorporated TDS software into their practice. The foregoing scenario not only illustrates the kind of benefits enjoyed by the practitioners and their patients; it also illustrates an adaptive approach for dealing with the array of available therapeutic support software. By identifying therapeutic information management problems within your practice and heeding the implementation imperatives noted above, you too can begin to realize the advantages offered by the wide range of TDS software available today.

6

PATIENT EDUCATION

Robert Hayward, MD; and Gary Kahn, MD, MEd

. . . .

Clinicians are under increasing pressure to educate patients, involve them in decision making, foster autonomy, and share responsibility for effective prevention, diagnosis, and treatment of health problems. At the same time, economic constraints continue to favor patient visits of short duration, and reimbursement schemes rarely compensate clinicians for the time needed to fully enable shared decision making. Moreover, as the focus of health care shifts toward disease prevention and health promotion, clinicians will be called on increasingly to foster behavioral and lifestyle modifications in their patients. This potentially time-consuming effort can be supported by new tools to facilitate efficient gathering and documenting of health history and preference assessment data. With or without these data-gathering tools, physicians also need systems to effectively educate patients and actively encourage their participation in health care. The following scenario illustrates how patient education programs can facilitate patient care.

Computerized Patient Education: A Clinical Scenario

You are relieved to find that the last patient in your busy morning clinic is a previously well, 47-year-old woman with acute dysuria. The history, physical examination, and urinalysis are straightforward. You quickly arrange appropriate treatment and remind your assistant to generate patient-information sheets about urinary tract infections generally and the antibiotic specifically.

On her way out the door, your patient asks whether she should have a "breast x-ray." Her menstrual periods stopped 6 months ago; she has never had cervical, ovarian, uterine, breast, bone, or cardiovascular problems, but her mother had a mastectomy at age 55 for breast cancer. Your patient observes that her friend has just started taking "female hormones," and she wonders whether she should too. You tell her that you had planned to advise screening mammography starting at age 50 but add that this would be a good time to reconsider her health risks and preventive care needs. She can extend today's visit by engaging in a computerized patient education session, using two interactive, guideline-based programs. One concerns general preventive care needs, and the other focuses on hormone-replacement therapy. Pleased to learn that she can deal with her questions immediately, your patient agrees to use the software, review customized educational printouts, and return next week to formulate a personal breast cancer prevention and estrogen prophylaxis program.

At the scheduled health maintenance visit, you review results of the automated health risk and preference questionnaires stored in your electronic medical record (EMR). The system documents and alerts you about unique risks that may justify mammographic screening at an earlier age than generally recommended. This information will come in handy because your patient's health insurer questions using screening mammography before age 50. The system also highlights expected benefits and harms from hormone prophylaxis as they apply to your patient's unique circumstances. After discussing your patient's reactions to her personalized printouts, you request a mammogram and prescribe estrogen for short-term relief of vaginal dryness while deferring a decision about long-term estrogen because of patient concerns about breast cancer risks.

Although information systems that enable this scenario exist today, they are new, hard to find, and difficult to integrate with existing EMR systems. Moreover, they are largely untested in typical clinical environments. Nonetheless, as the need for these capabilities grows, systems will improve and proliferate. For now, a number of computer-based products are available to support a systematic approach to patient education. In this chapter, we classify and describe patient-centered information systems and offer suggestions to help you begin using such tools in your practice.

HOW CAN PATIENT EDUCATION SOFTWARE HELP ME IN MY PRACTICE?

Improved patient education can benefit a practice in many ways. Generally speaking, informed patients tend to be satisfied patients. They are more likely to comply with health interventions, and they enjoy better outcomes. Health services research has shown that systematic patient education is associated with several specific kinds of benefits:

- Higher likelihood of adhering to medication regimen
- Longer persistence of behavior modification
- Shorter postoperative recovery times
- Better use of health care resources.

Quite apart from such improvements in the processes and outcomes of health care, consistently applied and well-documented patient education programs may reduce legal liability and improve recruitment and retention of patients in a practice.

Effective patient education programs can be tough

to implement and sustain. First, it is difficult to find appropriate educational materials. Further, impediments include insufficient time to teach the system to staff members and to administer the material to patients, lack of space for storing and organizing educational aids, and the high cost of many systems. Some barriers can be overcome by using structured educational interventions to reduce training, staff time, administration, storage, and organizational burdens.

Systematic Patient Education

Although nothing can replace the primacy of direct, personalized patient instruction by a knowledgeable and empathic physician, many practitioners supplement their verbal teachings with handouts, brochures, and instruction lists. Indeed, many clinics are equipped with posters and pamphlets giving information about common health problems and about self-help, teaching, and support groups. Larger clinics may maintain a collection of books, audiocassettes, videos, and playback equipment that patients can borrow. Waiting room delays can be sweetened with easy-to-read health periodicals, newsletters, and bulletin boards. Television monitors showing cable, satellite, or videocassette health promotion programs can accommodate a broad range of literacy levels.

Much of this sort of education, however, is hit-and-miss. Patients must correctly recognize their information needs, match those needs to relevant resources based on valid evidence, discern what does not apply to them, and follow through with indicated actions. A well-trained health educator can assess clinic objectives and patient needs, match materials to persons, monitor patient comprehension, and record attitudinal, behavioral, and health outcomes. But few practices could support such a professional. For most practices, however, computer-based patient education programs could enhance patients' access to meaningful resources, priming them for more satisfying, effective, and efficient clinician instruction and more durable results from that instruction.

A systematic patient education program is characterized by clear objectives and explicitly selected content and delivery methods. Such a program includes documentation of who is exposed to what and offers feedback about changes in patient feelings, actions, and health. A superior patient education system emulates good doctor-patient communication through individualization at the level of both the patient and the doctor. This type of system responds to the particular needs of individual patients, and it also accommodates the particular preferences of individual clinicians. Later in this chapter, we offer guides for selecting resources to help you achieve your patient education objectives.

Computer-enhanced Patient Education

In recent years, physicians have begun using personal computers to generate patient handouts about prescription medications, procedures, discharge instructions, and rehabilitation protocols. Approaches to patient-computer interaction continue to evolve in content, style, and interface. In content, the approach has evolved from, for example, informally worded messages to ones that are based on sound evidence and expressed using words that have been clinically tested for comprehensibility, reliability, and acceptability; in style, simple drill-and-practice techniques have evolved to the application of complex decision models; and regarding interface to the user, simple character-based computer terminals are giving way to interactive multimedia and hand-held devices. Newer systems facilitate provider- and patient-specific views of educational materials, with instructional methods and products adjusted to patient literacy and preferences. Most recently, patient education systems have begun to merge with other health care information systems such as drug information databases, emergency care systems, and EMRs.

Automated patient education systems offer many advantages over conventional, paper-based systems. They are easier to update and maintain. Electronic media permit frequent and rapid enhancement of entire libraries of materials. It is much easier to replace computer-based files and print current handouts as needed than to reacquire, reproduce, refile, and reintroduce updated, printed materials.

A related advantage of automated systems is almost instantaneous retrieval of a practically limitless inventory that otherwise would overwhelm cabinets, drawers, and display surfaces. Large volumes of electronically stored information can be moved rapidly using magnetic media or networks. Indeed, a rapidly growing collection of patient instruction materials now appears on the information superhighway (Internet), allowing clinicians and patients to rapidly obtain the most recent version of available documents on an as-needed basis from distant sites. Conventional printed materials tend to be more cumbersome to distribute, and their content is relatively static and inflexible. Electronically distributed educational materials can also be reconfigured and redeployed (within the limits of copyright) for use in new applications or for output in new formats (print, voice, video, or computer monitor). Many of the newer computer outputs match or exceed the level of graphic quality of paper publications.

The major disadvantages of computer-based patient education systems pertain to the same hardware capabilities that confer advantages. Hardware failures can cause the instant disappearance of all storage, retrieval, transport, and updating gains. Reliable hardware and network systems can be expensive to install. Finding adequate and appropriate space for a computer workstation can challenge many clinics, and, although the information in the computer is easily moved, the machine usually is not. Even when space is available, the time required to teach clinic staff, patients, or both, about the computer system may seem excessive, particularly while a system is being integrated into office routines and patients seek help using new programs.

Two Types of Patient Education Software

Software for patient instruction and education can be broadly classified according to whether it is interactive or not. While someone, of course, has to interact with the computer to make something happen, the focus here is on whether the patient interacts directly with the computer and, by so doing, affects the nature and content of the computer-aided learning. Noninteractive systems are widely available for creating, storing, and printing computer-generated patient handouts. Patient-interactive systems have proved their worth in research settings and are now increasingly available to clinicians. Interactive software can be subdivided according to whether the interaction is controlled by the patient or is directed, in large part, by the computer using predefined rules. Both types of computer-based patient education are described below.

Noninteractive Systems: Computer-generated Patient Handouts

Most patients remember less than half of what they hear from a physician. Verbal instructions about diagnostic tests and treatment plans are particularly vulnerable—if a patient forgets a key point, care could suffer. For this reason, many clinicians give patients written reminders in addition to the cryptic instructions that appear on drug prescriptions. Few physicians have the time to create, store, retrieve, duplicate, and update patient handouts to cover even their most common diagnoses, treatments, and rehabilitation protocols. Even without time constraints, few of us are trained to prepare clear patient educational material that strikes the right compromise between completeness and usability, accuracy and simplicity. The work of others can help. Many excellent instructional brochures are available from medical societies (for example, the American Lung Association); government agencies (for example, the Agency for Health Care Policy and Research); periodicals (for example, tear-outs); pharmaceutical companies (for example, audiocassettes about nicotine patch use); and medical suppliers. Once pro-

cured, however, these must be indexed, stored, retrieved, copied, and dispensed, and they are not easily modified to suit the special circumstances of your practice.

The simplest computer-generated patient handout (CGPH) systems handle much of the clerical work. They gather a set of stylistically consistent instruction sheets into an easily manipulated electronic collection, which can be printed individually or in sets, and they can be indexed, searched, and updated as the need arises. Older systems print simple text, while newer systems use the graphical capabilities of modern printers to mix text with pictures, diagrams, and a highlighted "bottom line." Pharmacists have been quick to acquire such systems. You may have noticed increasingly sophisticated medication instruction sheets given to your patients. Similarly, pressure to reduce length of stay for diagnostic and surgical procedures is leading same-day surgery units to use computer-generated discharge instructions because postoperative patients are particularly likely to misperceive or forget instructions. Computer-generated reminders improve follow-up compliance after discharge from emergency departments, another environment in which time and circumstance conspire to help patients forget key information.

More sophisticated CGPH systems allow the health provider to customize the handout before printing. For example, the patient's name, physician's name, date of visit, and supplementary notes can be added to a handout before it is printed. Less common are systems that offer full control over the content of messages, allowing some patients to be spared certain details and others to receive their physician's enhancement of a standard educational message. Customization can even extend to printing messages in more than one language or for more than one reading level.

Interactive Systems: Computer-based Patient Education

When teaching rather than reminding is the primary objective, interactive systems that involve the patient directly with a computer can be more helpful than a handout alone. In interactive systems, information is presented to the patient by the computer, which records and responds to the patient's response to that information. Patient comprehension can be assessed before proceeding to the next topic. In this way, interactive systems adapt the educational process to the patient's unique knowledge, comprehension, interests, and learning style. Simpler systems leave the patient in complete control of the educational experience. Patients determine the pace and pathway of teaching, with options to repeat, explore, or seek more detail. No penalty is given for going slow, and no reminder of the busy practitioner's time pressures is necessary. Indeed, putting patients in control of the educational process primes their interest in behavioral change and compliance.

More complex interactive systems use the analytic capabilities of the computer to gather and study information from patients and then use it to decide which educational materials to present and how. The patient still sets the pace of educational exchange, but the program uses available data to identify material most relevant to the patient's unique clinical situation. Systems are now available that can determine, for example, that women who have had a hysterectomy should receive different messages about the risks and benefits of hormone-replacement therapy than women who have not had a hysterectomy.

Computer-based patient education (CBPE) has been shown to significantly improve patient knowledge about risks for coronary disease, protection from sexually transmitted diseases, medication purpose and use, the basic pathophysiology of diabetes, and how to collect a "clean-catch" urine sample. In addition to improving knowledge, CBPE has also documented positive change in disease-related behaviors among patients with chronic illnesses such as diabetes and arthritis. Patients with chronic diseases are especially well suited for CBPE because they need to understand a good deal of complex information and translate that information into improved self-care skills, a time- and resource-intensive task which often overwhelms the provider's capacity to do it properly. For potentially embarrassing topics such as sexually transmitted diseases, dysthymia, and substance-abuse screening, patients have been shown to prefer computer interaction to face-to-face interviews.

Besides improving patient behavior and patient knowledge about disease processes and outcomes, other advantages of interactive CBPE include:

- Availability when live instructors are busy or absent

- Consistency and patience in gathering and dispensing information

- Customized instruction

- Patient privacy and avoidance of embarrassment

- Apt use of feedback and reinforcement
- Precise documentation of the learning process and outcome.

The success of CBPE is enhanced by a user-friendly and unintimidating patient-computer interface. For example, an osteoarthritis program for elderly patients uses just a few color-coded data-entry keys, large computer screen fonts, and a simple online-help system. Case simulation and games can engage patient concentration. Patients with diabetes, for example, can use interactive programs to learn how to administer insulin.

Special devices have been developed to optimize the reliability and validity of patient-computer interaction. For example, the HealthQuiz computer is a four-button, battery-powered video device on which health questions are read and answered by a patient before customized feedback is generated for the patient and the clinician. Like a laptop video game, it has an exceptionally simple user interface and is easily moved from one patient to another. Other portable interfaces will appear as palmtop and pen-based computers penetrate health care computing and become more durable and less costly.

Patient-computer interaction does not have to occur in the office. In France, a diabetes CBPE and monitoring system which used teletext terminals and telephone connections improved patients' dietary habits and reduced blood hemoglobin A_{1c} and fructosamine levels. Some health maintenance organizations use computerized telephone questionnaires to help patients make appropriate appointments and adhere to preventive care recommendations.

A common objection to CBPE is that patients may resent sharing personal information with and receiving health suggestions from a machine. Studies as far back as the mid-1960s, however, consistently show the opposite. Patients value any intervention that they expect to improve their physician's knowledge about their health. Indeed, patients today may legitimately wonder why their physicians do not make better use of computers when the advantages offered by these devices are everywhere else in evidence. Errors in recording and recalling patient information are increasingly difficult to abide when one can walk up to any banking machine and reliably control personal transactions on the other side of the world. Health services research has shown that patients welcome computer-assisted care as an enhancement, not a replacement, of individualized health care, and this acceptance crosses age, education, and socioeconomic boundaries.

WHAT COMPUTERIZED PATIENT EDUCATION PROGRAMS ARE CURRENTLY AVAILABLE?

At present, the most common computerized patient instruction tools are noninteractive and are widely available, compatible with a full range of computer operating systems, and relatively easy to integrate with existing office systems. Interactive programs are rapidly improving, but many still require dedicated equipment for patient-computer sessions and can be difficult to blend with existing systems and office routines. Several selected patient education software products are listed in Table 6-1; this listing along with the discussion below should serve as a starting point for identifying available products and evaluating their potential utility in your practice.

Noninteractive Programs

Office-generated Handouts

Available technology allows you to manage CGPHs in various ways. The most direct is to write your own handouts, using a word processor. You

Table 6-1. Patient Education Products Discussed

Product	Platform	Price*	Publisher or Manufacturer	Address	Phone and Fax Numbers
AskAdvice	Windows	$-$$	First DataBank	1111 Bayhill Drive, Suite 350 San Bruno, CA 94066	Tel: 415-588-5454 Fax: 415-588-4003
Computerized Lifestyle Assessment	DOS	$$	Multi-Health Systems, Inc.	908 Niagara Falls Boulevard North Tonawanda, NY 14120	Tel: 800-456-3003 Fax: 416-424-1736
Dr. Welford's Chart Notes	DOS	$$$-$$$$	MEDCOM Information Systems	2117 Stonington Avenue Hoffman Estates, IL 60195	Tel: 800-424-0258 Fax: 708-885-1591
Electronic Drug Reference 6.0	DOS 3.0	$$ single user	Clinical Reference Systems, Ltd .	7100 East Belleview Avenue Suite 208 Greenwood Village, CO 80111-1636	Tel: 800-237-8401 303-220-1661 Fax: 303-220-1685
Health Probe	DOS, Windows	$$ single user	Healthcare Data	5311 Mt. Pleasant North Drive Greenwood, IN 46142	Tel: 317-887-1326 Fax: 317-887-1326
Mayo Clinic Family Health Book	Macintosh, Windows	$$ single user	IVI Publishing	7500 Flying Cloud Drive Minneapolis, MN 55435	Tel: 800-432-1332
Medication Adviser 5.0	DOS 3.0	$$ single user	Clinical Reference Systems, Ltd.	7100 East Belleview Avenue Suite 208 Greenwood Village, CO 80111-1636	Tel: 800-237-8401 303-220-1661 Fax: 303-220-1685
Prevent	HealthQuiz Computer	N/A	Nellcor, Inc.	Clinical Information Systems 4280 Hacienda Drive Pleasanton, CA 94588	Tel: 510-463-4225 Fax: 510-463-4594
Shared Decision-Making Programs	Interactive videodisks	$$$-$$$$	Foundation for Informed Medical Decision Making	P.O. Box 5457 Hanover, NH 03755	Tel: 603-650-1180 Fax: 603-650-1125
SuperDOC!	DOS	$$	SuperDOC! Software	P.O. Box 1113 Harrisonburg, VA 22801	Tel: 800-541-0322 Fax: 703-433-7731

* $ = under $100; $$ = $101 to $500; $$$ = $501 to $1000; $$$$ = over $1000. Prices are approximate at the time of printing.

may already own a word processor, and using it to make your own informative handouts affords maximum control over content and format. You can prepare outlines, which are then used as templates to be modified as needed for different groups of patients. Graphical additions can be as simple as a logo for your practice or as complex as pictures illustrating procedures. Carefully consider the reading level of your handouts, as patient comprehension is critical. The sort of grammar checker now commonly packaged with word processors can help with this task. Indeed, translator programs can also do a rough first draft of your handout in another language (make sure the result is edited by someone fluent in the language). Depending on your word processor and the rest of your computer configuration, you may be able to rapidly print a handout using a few simple keystrokes or mouse clicks.

Database programs can also be used to create your own CGPH system. Newer versions can accommodate large text fields, which could contain the content of your handouts, and form-generating utilities, which can be used to give printouts an attractive appearance. Databases allow you to retrieve handouts by searching keyword indexes. If you have a scheduling or medical record program running on your system, you can create links or macros to automatically attach patient identifiers to any handout you print—a nice touch.

An obvious drawback of self-generated handouts is that you have a lot of writing and typing to do. If you already have a set of favorite brochures, you can speed transcription by bringing that material into your word processing files with a scanner and optical character recognition (OCR) software. To avoid the start-up costs and labor of doing this properly, you can have a desktop publishing service bureau do the scanning work for about $1 to $3 per page (versus $300+ for a hand-held or $800+ for a flatbed scanner, and $400+ for good OCR software). You must also consider copyright restrictions when incorporating such materials for redistribution.

Commercially Produced Handouts

What commercial CGPH programs may lack, owing to their practice-independent content, they make up for with volume and breadth of content. Better developers subject their content to systematic testing for comprehensibility and patient acceptability after ensuring that the messages are based on sound evidence. Good programs also allow control over the appearance of actual printouts, including the ability to edit existing handouts and create new handouts or add additional ones from your own collection. Many practices will appreciate the increasing number of programs that allow printing in more than one language and reading level. Of course, you need to invest time initially to review and possibly edit or delete handouts that conflict with the advice you are comfortable giving. You do not want computer-generated messages to cause your patients confusion and concern.

The most common CGPH programs deal with medication issues for a variety of compelling reasons: the prevalence of patient noncompliance and drug errors; the interests of pharmaceutical companies; concerns about increasing numbers of medication-related malpractice lawsuits; pharmacy-based experience with and development of CGPH software; and the wide availability of relatively good drug information databases, which allow patient instruction systems to be integrated with provider information systems.

Figure 6-1. Adult Health Advisor. Top. General topical index, with contact dermatitis highlighted. **Bottom.** Screen showing the beginning of the handout on contact dermatitis.

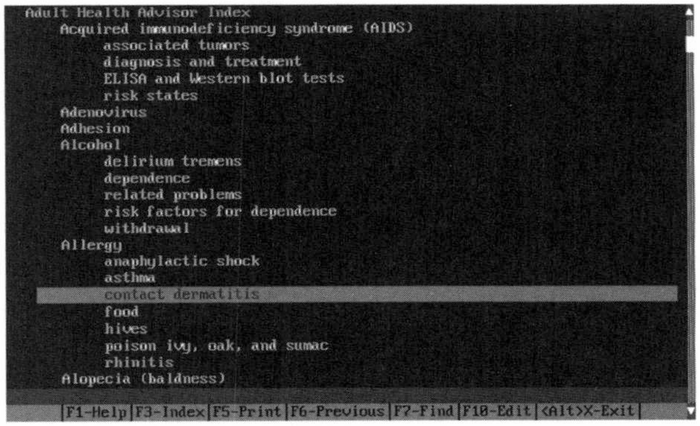

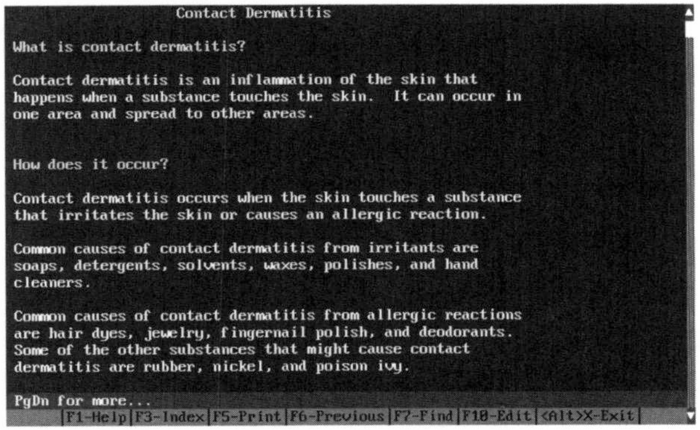

For example, AskAdvice generates medication handouts derived from the *USP DI* (Drug Information for the Patients, U.S. Pharmacopoeial Convention, Inc.). AskAdvice can run alongside a companion program, AskRx Plus, which uses the same Windows-based software environment to provide the clinician with drug information and interactions from the *USP DI* (volume for health professionals). Within AskAdvice, patient details (name, address, age, and so on); provider information (name, address, telephone number, and so on); and personalized instructions can be incorporated in the handout. The provider can control the type of drug information printed in the handout (for example, you may want to delete pregnancy warnings for male patients), and the printer font size can be adjusted to help the visually impaired. AskAdvice does not allow you to edit the wording or content of actual drug information for the patient.

Two programs from Clinical Reference Systems, Ltd. (CRS)—Medication Adviser and Electronic Drug Reference—perform similar functions on computers running DOS. In addition to providing medication handouts, CRS also offers automated patient handout packages for general adult health, pediatrics, and obstetrics and gynecology (Figure 6-1). So far, it is not possible to search across all packages simultaneously. Other companies also combine libraries of different types of patient handouts, and the trend favors integration of handout packages with general clinical information systems. For example, Dr. Welford's Chart Notes is an EMR system developed by a general internist that automates and integrates various functions—prescription writing, health advice, procedural instructions, and any other handouts that a user may wish to add—with an EMR and other administrative and decision support tools. Indeed, these sorts of capabilities are sufficiently important that you should look for them before buying a new office information system (*see* Chapters 1 and 2).

Another approach taken by programs such as Super Doc! focuses on emergency department discharge and assembles relevant documents from within a single program. Handouts concerning the patient's diagnosis, treatment, self-care, and follow-up can be printed along with prescriptions, work or school permission slips, form letters to third-party insurers, and consultation requests. A copy of the printed material can be signed and kept with the chart as a record of discharge instruction. Theoretically, these programs could be used not only in emergency departments but in office practice as well.

Other Sources of Information for Patients

Overlap can be found among the programs that physicians might use to educate patients and the programs that patients can access themselves or through other professional sources such as pharmacists or managed care organizations. Some of these programs are mentioned below and in the next section (*see under* Interactive Programs).

An increasing array of information useful for patient education may also be accessed on Internet. Examples of such material include the Medical College of Wisconsin's International Travelers Clinic, the New York State Education and Research Network Breast Cancer Information Clearing House, and the National Cancer Institute's patient information sheets. (The online addresses of these Internet resources are given in the Appendix.) Although such information can currently be accessed free of charge, the user must invest time in accessing, evaluating, and preparing this information for patient use. As more and more patient groups use online systems for communication and information exchange, the quantity and quality of this material will likely increase.

Another strategy for bringing health information to patients' homes had a prototype in Harvard Community Health Plan's outpatient facility in Burlington, Massachusetts. Software developed by InterPractice Systems integrated EMRs, clinical decision support systems, administrative and financial systems, and a patient education system. The latter allowed patients to access information and advice using a personal computer and modem, 24 hours a day. By interacting with an electronic triage system, patients could discern trivial from significant symptoms, monitor chronic health problems (for example, hypertension and asthma), and provide health-risk information before preventive visits. A result of the exchange could have been self-care instructions or an automatically arranged appointment with a clinician. All interactions were recorded in the patient's medical record. Other managed care organizations are also experimenting with this type of patient interaction.

Interactive Programs

Earlier in this chapter, we made a distinction between interactive software that is controlled by the patient and that which is directed by the computer. This distinction does injustice to some programs that have both patient- and computer-directed components but highlights different ways of matching content to need. The most rudimentary patient-directed systems use the computer as an electronic page turner. A corpus of educational material is broken up into small parts that can be presented on the screen sequentially. Patients determine the speed with which they progress through educational material, and they limit the amount of information read in a single session.

More sophisticated systems use a branching and looping architecture for determining the sequence in which instructional units are presented. Patients take a unique path through the information, determined by selections from menus of options. A variation on this theme has patients answer questions. Depending on the answer, the learner embarks on different paths, reviewing the points missed, moving ahead, exploring in more depth, or switching to another topic altogether.

The basic structure of a patient-directed computer interaction can be used with different methods of presenting content. Older systems rely entirely on text messages displayed on a computer screen. Newer, CD-ROM–based products such as the Mayo Clinic Family Health Book allow patients to browse through articles that are illustrated with color diagrams, digitized photographs, sound clips, and even video clips. Although multimedia glitz often pleases the senses enough to distract from poorly organized and validated content, some recent systems tether multimedia technology to valid content and sound educational methods. They achieve a potent medium for patient education. Among such systems are the interactive videodisks developed by the Foundation for Informed Medical Decision Making in Dartmouth, New Hampshire. This approach uses interactive video technology (a computer-controlled laser disc player with touch-screen display) to help patients make informed decisions based on an engaging review of high-quality information available from outcomes research. The videodisks are rich with patient and clinician interviews, allowing learners to tap this source of experience as well. The first of these programs (known as shared decision-making programs or SDPs) concerned management of benign prostatic hyperplasia and the risks and benefits of surgical and nonsurgical treatment. Since 1989, one test site using this program has witnessed a 44% reduction in surgery, with cost savings of $170 000 to $200 000 per year. Four similar programs from the foundation are in widespread use, and several others are under development. A screen from a newer SDP is shown in Figure 6-2. The programs are licensed for approximately $1000 per year, and the interactive video system needed to play the SDPs costs from $6000 to $8000. The foundation is exploring methods other than videodisk to disseminate the content of the SDPs.

Computer-directed interactive patient education systems go to greater lengths to gather, analyze, and apply patient-reported data in order to configure a

Figure 6-2. Screen from a shared decision-making program. Provides patients with information on risks and benefits of hormone-replacement therapy.

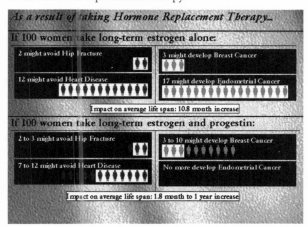

personalized educational experience. This type of software underwent extensive development over a decade ago, when health risk assessment programs became popular. These programs gathered personal, family, and lifestyle information from patients, and some combined the data with clinical variables such as cholesterol, blood pressure, and height and weight. The programs then applied the data to epidemiologic models to generate feedback for patients about the likely effect of their risks and behaviors on longevity and well-being. Unfortunately, predictions made by these programs have not proved especially accurate. Modern versions of risk assessment software concern themselves less with predictions and more with encouraging healthy lifestyles through

personalized, meaningful educational messages. An excellent example is Computerized Lifestyle Assessment from Multi-Health Systems, Inc. Patients are guided through a health history and lifestyle questionnaire. The program then gives patients personalized feedback that teaches about preventable illness and highlights individual opportunities for preventing disease and promoting health.

Some programs gather information from patients to determine how clinical practice guidelines might apply and be used. Again, patients are guided through sophisticated branching questionnaires that gather information required by a particular guideline. The computer can respond to patient uncertainty and make the questioning experience efficient and fun. Information from the patient or clinician, or both, is then processed by algorithms and probabilistic decision models to prepare appropriate reminders for the clinician and personalized educational feedback for the patient. An example of this approach uses the HealthQuiz computer, a special patient-computer interface noted earlier in this chapter. Prevent is the name of a software application that runs on the HealthQuiz and Windows computers. Patients answer questions about their health, behaviors, family illnesses, interests, and preferences before guideline-compliant preventive care recommendations and educational patient feedback are prepared. The computer uses patient- and clinician-reported data and guideline-based algorithms to determine how feedback will be configured for individual patients. Both the HealthQuiz computer and Prevent software are marketed by Nellcor, Inc., which also sells other programs similar to Prevent.

Interactive computer simulations provide opportunities for patients to learn in the same context in which new knowledge is needed. For example, a person with diabetes may learn how to adjust his or her insulin by interacting with a simulation program that models the body's blood sugar and physiologic response to insulin dose, diet, and exercise. The complexity of the simulation can be controlled by the computer program, introducing more realistic scenarios as the learner progresses. Indeed, to further engage the patient, simulations can be run as games where entertainment, competition, and fantasy are used to enhance learning. Health Probe, from Healthcare Data, is an example of such an application. This type of software is increasingly prevalent on the shelves of general computer stores. You may wish to keep abreast of the more popular programs so that you can react appropriately should your patients ask questions about them.

HOW CAN I SUCCESSFULLY IMPLEMENT PATIENT EDUCATION SOFTWARE IN MY PRACTICE?

Earlier we said that a systematic approach to patient education is characterized by clear objectives, sound content, effective delivery methods, good records, and meaningful performance indicators. Here we offer guides to determine whether a particular software product is likely to become a valid, valuable, and usable component of your overall patient education strategy. In this context, validity refers to the accuracy of educational messages and the extent to which they are based on sound evidence. Value concerns the likely effect of the product on your practice, as judged by the frequency with which you encounter the problems targeted by the educational software; the need of your patients for education in this area; the degree to which those needs are unmet; and the expected health, administrative, and economic benefits from meeting those needs. Usability reflects how much work you must do to successfully implement the software.

Unfortunately, it is problematic to rely exclusively on present-day software reviews to deal specifically with issues of validity, value, and usability. Because many reviews do not explore these issues comprehensively and software products often change rapidly, we strongly urge you to do your own evaluation. For this, you must obtain demonstration versions of the programs that interest you. We suggest that you make a short-list of programs of a type you find appealing, for which you have the necessary equipment (hardware, operating system, storage capacity), and in which you would consider investing. Remember to consider not only the original software installation but also the cost of updates, license renewals, and anticipated equipment upgrades. (The previous section of this chapter along with the Introduction to this book offer suggestions for identifying potentially useful software and may help provide a starting point for your list.) Then draft a form letter to vendors requesting information about the evidence base for the educational materials and any proof of comprehensibility (in order to assess its validity). Ask what topics are covered, how they are dealt with, and whether the program is interactive or noninteractive, patient-directed or computer-directed (to assess value and sophistication); and get particulars about how the software works and may interact with other programs you use (to assess usability). Demonstration programs are usually available. The best demos are fully functioning versions of a program that are somehow "crippled" by an expiration date, limited number of uses, or inability to store or print information. If the vendor will not provide a demonstration program, she or he should at least give you the name of a customer in your area so that you can visit and observe the software in action. Attention to this detail will help familiarize you with the idiosyncrasies (some of them annoying) inherent in all types of software.

Software Selection Guides

With the software in front of you, try to answer the following questions to assess the validity, value, and usability of the program.

Validity

What is the educational content? Are handouts sufficiently detailed? Some drug information packages, for example, take shortcuts by providing general informa-

tion about a class of drugs (for example, beta-blockers) in place of specific items (for example, sotalol).

Where does content come from? How were patient education or instruction messages generated, by whom, and based on what evidence?

When was the content last reviewed for accuracy and completeness?

How is content delivered? Has this strategy been tested with patients like yours to assess its comprehensibility, acceptability, and reliability? What evidence is available that the product accomplishes its educational goals?

Value

Will patients value this program? Is the educational content of a type that is important and that your patients do not already get in an acceptable manner from another source?

Will staff value this program? Will the software ease staff burdens, or will it add to them? How will you integrate the software products with your current work flow and documentation systems?

Will external reviewers value this program? Will it produce output that will improve your charting abilities, facilitate third-party payment for services, or show up well on a practice audit? Can you keep a legally valid log of which patient got which handout or other educational intervention?

Will you value this program? Can you correlate software use with changes in patient behaviors, health outcomes, practice costs, patient recruitment, or retention? Does the system generate periodic performance reports? How much will it cost you to keep the system running? Will you be charged for support, updates, enhancements, or bug fixes? If the program integrates many functions, how much do you save by not having to buy other software?

Usability

How will clinicians interact with the software? Can you easily seek and find patient education materials by keyword or other search strategies? Can print-outs be customized? If so, is this a straightforward process? Can you add your own handouts to the library? Do you use your own word processor, which is familiar to you, or must you learn a custom text editor?

How will patients interact with the software? Is special hardware needed, or will you need to dedicate a computer and kiosk for patient use? For computer interaction, do patients use a keyboard (least desirable); or a pointing device such as a mouse, pen, trackball, or joystick (more desirable); or is almost no tool required, as with a touch-screen, voice-activation, or custom interface (most desirable)? Is the interface intuitive and "guessable"? Is there a simple online help system? Can the interface accommodate different languages and reading levels? Are handouts simple, appealing, and printed with large fonts?

How will systems interact with the software? Can the product function as well on a network as on a stand-alone computer? Does the software multitask, that is, allow for multiple programs to be open at once? Can information such as patient name and related data be moved easily between programs? Are security measures in place to prevent patients and staff from intentionally (hackers!) or unintentionally reading, damaging, or deleting confidential patient data or other files or programs on the system?

Implementing Patient Education Software

Installation of a patient education system demands new work skills from clinical staff and therefore must follow adequate consultation with them. All clinicians in your practice should be familiar with all of the content that could be generated by an automated information handout or interactive education system. You should make sure that this information is consistent with your clinical practices and be prepared to either modify the content if discrepancies exist or have a plan to inform patients of your perspective. You should consider the effect that the information will have on each patient to whom you dispense it. For example, will patients with multiple nonorganic somatic complaints be likely to experience all the side effects on your medication handout? Similarly, you should be ready to respond to questions that the educational programs might provoke, such as "how likely am I to experience this serious side effect mentioned in the medication handout?" Indeed, this process of reviewing patient education software programs could breathe new life into your continuing education and in-service programs. Enlisting support and enthusiasm from your staff increases the likelihood that the new software and office routines will work smoothly.

As a logistic matter, you need to consider who will do what in getting handouts to patients. By asking the office team to work with a demonstration program and pretest the software, you may learn unanticipated lessons. It may become clear, for example, that a dedicated workstation and work area for management of patient handouts is necessary and that the receptionist, not the doctor or nurse, should organize the handouts at presentation to or departure from the office. You may discover that an interactive educational program triggers patient concerns and so should be administered before a physician encounter, allowing you to review important points at the visit.

As you discover what details and concerns must be addressed for successful implementation in your practice, you are certain to experience why computer-facilitated patient education is rapidly becoming a potent aid for the clinician as well as a valuable resource for the patient. As the applications of computers to patient education are proliferating and changing at a bewildering rate, you will need to keep pace with the evolving technology. To keep up, you need to track not only software marketed to physicians but also a rapidly growing library of educational and self-help titles sold directly to the public. A better informed public can be a healthier public.

7

Personal Continuing Medical Education

Edward P. Hoffer, MD, FACP

. . . .

How can computer-based continuing medical education help me?

We are all aware of the explosion in biomedical knowledge that has made much of what we learned in medical school incomplete or outdated. These circumstances have only reinforced the need for all conscientious physicians to be lifelong students who never stop learning about new diagnostic and therapeutic strategies. Traditionally, continuing medical education (CME) has been done by reading journals and attending postgraduate courses, as well as by informal one-on-one learning from colleagues and consultants. The personal computer offers us a new tool for our continuing education, one with many theoretical and some demonstrated advantages.

Who Should Pursue Computer-based Education?

If you enjoy using computers and find yourself using them now for things you used to do by hand, such as writing checks or keeping your daily schedule, you will probably enjoy much of the computer-based CME that is now available. If you want to begin using your office computer for something beyond billing, you may find educational software an easy way to begin. In addition, if you find getting enough CME credits to be a problem or resent having to take days away from the office to attend a course, you may be ready to take the plunge.

If, on the other hand, you are a subspecialist whose major CME interests lie in keeping up with your subspecialty, then you may have difficulty finding material specifically suited to your needs, although such programs are appearing more frequently. Also, if you are currently satisfied with the scope and depth of your CME activities, you may be less likely to see a major benefit from computer-based CME. However, the newer generation of multimedia programs featuring rich clinical case presentations and discussions are probably worth the attention of all clinicians.

What Is Different about Computer-based Education?

The usual CME program consists of a lecture or series of lectures, which must be aimed at the "average" attendee. Thus, some in the audience may be bored by hearing material that is already familiar, while others may find the pace too rapid. Furthermore, the lecture format makes it difficult to actively engage audiences in the learning process, which is problematic since learning tends to be greater when learners participate. A well-designed computer program, on the other hand, allows users to overcome the potential disadvantages of the traditional lecture format.

First, computer-based CME tends to be highly interactive, providing the user with some information and then eliciting a user response to a query based on that information. Using these programs, the learner is allowed to proceed at his or her own pace, taking as much time as needed to cover the material. In addition, the computer-based format overcomes the limitations of the "linear" lecture format, where all attendees are exposed to the same material in the same order. With computer-based learning, the user easily controls not only the order in which different topics are covered but also the depth to which they are covered. Appropriately designed programs allow users who are new to a topic to focus on the basics, while those more familiar with the material can choose to concentrate more on finer points or on self-assessment. Commercial computer-based CME programs vary widely in the extent to which the user can create a custom-tailored CME program.

The Value of Computer-based CME

Another potential issue with traditional CME is cost. To gain the required CME credits, physicians frequently take time away from their practice to attend postgraduate CME courses, which usually involves course fees and may also include the cost of transportation to and lodging at the course site. Even greater is the indirect cost of time lost from your practice. Of course, many hospitals and universities offer "free" opportunities to obtain CME credits, but these offerings may not meet all of your educational needs. Computer-based CME programs begin to approximate the breadth and depth of coverage typically found in postgraduate courses. The growing collection of computer-based CME products offers an increasingly attractive and convenient option for addressing at least some of your needs for continuing education and CME credits.

Most of the educational products described in this chapter offer American Medical Association (AMA) Category 1 CME credits. The number of hours available for use of each program varies from 3 to 6 or more. The publisher usually requires you to take a post-test to claim the hours and get your certificate. The specifics about CME credit are generally listed in advertisements. If no mention is made, you can probably assume that Category 1 credit is not offered.

Patient Problem Solving and CME

Using the medical literature or databases or other authoritative resources for addressing clinical problems arising during patient care is an important component of continuing education. In fact, such activity can be used to earn Category 2 credits toward AMA's Physician Recognition Award. The computer environment not only allows the user to search readily for knowledge related to patient care but also theoretically permits the searching activity and results to be recorded for CME reporting and self-assessment purposes.

Some Canadian physicians are already using computer-based systems to document and report their continuing professional development activities within the Maintenance of Competence, or MOCOMP, Program (*see* Appendix, Chapter 7). This program enables physicians to track the types of questions that arise in their practice, the results of their search for answers, and the effect of this search on their practice. The MOCOMP diary is also used to record other CME activities and thus enables physicians to track their professional development activities while also enabling the Royal College of Physicians and Surgeons of Canada to officially recognize this development.

The growing value placed on practice-based learning activities is evidenced by the AMA Category 2 CME credit requirements and by the MOCOMP Program. Fortunately, such learning suggests a natural link between the types of programs discussed in this chapter and the question-answering technologies discussed in most of the other chapters in this book. If this trend continues, users can expect (or perhaps should demand) that medical software developers routinely provide MOCOMP diary-like front-ends on their products to enable users to track, report, and evaluate their practice-based learning activities.

Future Developments in Personal CME

Although many of the programs mentioned later in this chapter are distributed on diskettes, multimedia technology is shifting the spotlight onto CD-ROM. Multimedia CME programs using CD-ROM and related technologies are already beginning to offer audiovisual material such as full-motion video clips from lectures, angiograms, and audio from phonocardiograms. High-resolution graphics such as photographs of optic fundi and skin lesions, as well as radiographic imaging studies, can also be readily displayed for education and self-evaluation purposes. The breadth and sophistication of these multimedia educational programs should increase dramatically in the near term as program developers learn to make optimal use of this technology. In the not too distant future, this multimedia functionality will be readily available on the Internet.

Just past multimedia on the CME horizon lies "virtual reality." Virtual reality refers to the use of sophisticated computer simulations with realistic graphical images and is being used experimentally to create lifelike simulations of events such as diagnostic and surgical procedures (*see Medical World News, February 1994*). Within the next few years, virtual reality systems will probably be able to teach you endoscopy and other manual skills via the computer. However, such techniques will likely be used primarily at centralized learning centers for the foreseeable future because of the expensive equipment needed.

WHAT COMPUTER-BASED CME PRODUCTS ARE AVAILABLE NOW?

Available Media

Several options exist for accessing computer-based CME material, including through an online system and on floppy diskette, CD-ROM, or videodisk. Some individual programs such as DISCOTEST (floppy diskette and CD-ROM) and the RxDx series (floppy diskette and online) are available in more than one of these media. Obviously, each medium carries different implications for the cost, versatility, and other factors related to CME product use.

CD-ROM–based CME programs can exploit the power of multimedia but are usually more costly and require special hardware. Conversely, floppy-disk–based programs usually display only text but tend to be less expensive and require no additional equipment. Online systems such as US HealthLink allow

the user with a modem to sample CME programs such as RxDx for a modest online charge. Users with access to Internet and the World Wide Web via Mosaic (*see* Chapter 8) should keep an eye open for sophisticated, multimedia educational programs; the Virtual Hospital provides a glimpse of what those programs might look like. While videodisks have been used in institutional settings, they do not appear to be in widespread use elsewhere. CD-ROM and subsequent technologies will likely supplant the older videodisk technology.

Target Audience: The Generalist

Physician-oriented material for computer-aided instruction is now widely available. Most software is aimed at the generalist and primary-care physician. With limited exceptions, medical subspecialists, as noted earlier, will not find many useful programs in their field of expertise. Subspecialists can find educational value in the current software, however, by exploring areas outside of their specialty. Subject matter that is considered of wide interest often has computer-based instructional programs available from several sources. One obvious example is in the field of cardiopulmonary resuscitation; programs on cardiopulmonary resuscitation/advanced cardiac life support (CPR/ACLS) are available from at least four different publishers.

Functionality: Making Use of the Computer's Capacity

Less and less common, but still seen, is the use of the computer as a "page turner." Many of the early computer-based educational programs simply reproduced paper-based products on a screen. Since booklets are cheaper and more portable than computers, and since it is generally easier to read blocks of text from the printed page than from a screen, this type of program provides little advantage. The better computer-based programs use the computer to go beyond what can be done in the print medium, which may mean using sound, video, or graphics to illustrate a point or demonstrate a clinical finding or possibly presenting the user with a case simulation that provides different decision paths with consequent different outcomes in the same case. But in all cases, it means the authors have understood how best to use the medium; simply adding color screens and a mouse interface to blocks of text is not a substitute for rewriting material to use the computer effectively. Many current programs are relatively unsophisticated compared with what the technology can offer. Others are quite impressive and foreshadow a new generation of computer-based CME products.

Computer-based CME Materials on Diskette

The following paragraphs briefly describe several currently available educational programs that may be of interest to physicians. The prices and information on CME credit are given as a rough benchmark; readers are encouraged to contact the publishers listed here, consult the Appendix, and use the strategies discussed in the Introduction to identify specific programs likely to meet your needs. Information about the publishers of the programs noted here is listed in Table 7-1. (Note that the author of this chapter is the primary author of the RxDx series of programs published by Williams and Wilkins Electronic Media.)

Cardinal Health Systems

Cardinal Health Systems has published a series of 19 computer-based instructional programs under the global title of Cyberlog. Currently available titles include Inflammatory Arthritis; Thyroid Diseases; Fluid, Electrolytes and Acid-Base Balance; Acute Respiratory Failure; Management of Type II Diabetes Mellitus; Hypertension; Selected Environmental Emergencies; Coronary Artery Disease; Major Gastrointestinal Disorders; Prevention of Coronary Artery Disease; Inpatient Infectious Diseases; Outpatient Infectious Diseases; Clinical Pharmacology I; Sports Medicine: Injury and Treatment; Sports Medicine: Rehabilitation and Prevention; Arrhythmias; Congestive Heart Failure; Anxiety Disorders; and Cardiac Emergency Simulator.

CME credits are awarded for the Cyberlog programs for an extra fee of $15 to $20 per program. The list price for each title except the last is $99.95; if you buy four or more at one time, the price is $89.95 each. Cardiac Emergency Simulator sells for $149. Each program contains a tutorial, which uses text and graphics to introduce the subject, but they seem to be aimed at the neophyte and may be too introductory for many physicians.

A unique feature of Cyberlog is the inclusion in each program of Decision-Aid Tools—various calculation functions or table look-ups to help you in specific patient management situations. Each program

Table 7-1. Publishers of Computer-based Continuing Medical Education Materials Discussed

Publisher or Manufacturer	Address	Phone and Fax Numbers
BDR, Inc.	P.O. Box 812098 Wellesley, MA 02181-0013	Tel: 800-998-6374 617-237-4788 Fax: 617-239-0391
Cardinal Health Systems	4600 West 77th Street Suite 150 Edina, MN 55435	Tel: 800-328-0180 Fax: 612-835-7141
Challenger Corporation	5530 Summer Avenue Memphis, TN 38134	Tel: 800-676-0822 Fax: 901-385-8380
Continuing Medical Education Associates, Inc.	4015 Hancock Street Suite 120 San Diego, CA 92110	Tel: 800-227-2632 619-223-2997 Fax: 619-223-8854
Decker Electronic Publishing, Inc.	1 James Street South Hamilton, ON L8N 3K7 Canada	Tel: 800-568-7281 416-522-7016 Fax: 905-522-7839
Health Sciences Consortium	201 Silver Cedar Court Chapel Hill, NC 27514	Tel: 919-942-8731 Fax: 919-942-3689
HealthCare Information Services, Inc.	2335 American River Drive Suite 307 Sacramento, CA 95825	Tel: 800-468-1128 916-648-8075 Fax: 916-648-8078
IVI Publishing	7500 Flying Cloud Drive Minneapolis, MN 55435	Tel: 800-661-6170
Keyboard Publishing	482 Norristown Road Blue Bell, PA 19422	Tel: 800-945-4551 610-832-0945 Fax: 610-832-0948
Mosby-Yearbook, Inc.	11830 Westline Industrial Drive St. Louis, MO 63146-3318	Tel: 800-426-4545 Fax: 800-535-9935
Reuters Health Information Services, Inc.	6425 Powers Ferry Road, NW Suite 300 Atlanta, GA 30339	Tel: 800-797-2633 Fax: 404-988-8655
Scientific American Medicine	415 Madison Avenue New York, NY 10017	Tel: 800-545-0554 Fax: 212-980-3062
SilverPlatter Education, Inc.	100 River Ridge Road Norwood, MA 02062-5043	Tel: 800-343-0064 617-769-2599 Fax: 617-769-8763
Williams and Wilkins Electronic Media	428 East Preston Street Baltimore, MD 21202	Tel: 800-527-5597 Fax: 410-528-4422

also includes three to five short case studies to which you can apply the material covered in the tutorial as well as a printed text (generally running 64 pages) covering the material. This text is also available on disk with enhanced indexing. Many of the programs do not seem to have been recently updated; the copyright dates are mostly from 1989 or earlier. How important this factor is obviously varies by topic. A demonstration disk is available, listing all of the available titles and giving the table of contents, educational objectives, and author information for each. It also includes four short working "samples" from four different programs. Spending half an hour with this disk should give you a good feel for the programs. (Note that Cardinal is no longer updating or supporting these programs.)

Challenger Corporation

The Challenger Corporation offers MD-Challenger, a program consisting of about 4000 multiple-choice questions on all aspects of acute care medicine. The program is available for the Macintosh and IBM-PC (under either Windows or DOS) and is approved for up to 200 hours of Category 1 CME credit. While I would ordinarily dismiss a multiple-choice examination as a poor use of the computer, this one is different. The questions are all categorized by topic and indexed, and you can use them as a mini-textbook, with the correct answers and a brief discussion given. You can also call up references on each question or topic. A running tally is kept of your score both on the total examination and by subject, allowing you to

pinpoint weak areas. The price is rather high at $595, which includes 100 hours of CME credit and $150 for each additional 50 hours of CME credit up to 200 total hours. The demonstration I received included a "special limited-time offer" of $295 for the single-user version. How long this price will be available was not stated.

Decker Electronic Publishing, Inc.

Decker is the publisher of two specialty-oriented CME series. One, produced under the auspices of the American College of Obstetricians and Gynecologists (ACOG), is titled Programs in Clinical Decision Making and is aimed at the obstetrics-gynecology specialist. The price varies from $140 per year for ACOG junior fellows to $350 per year for nonmembers and is for a six-issue series, published bimonthly. This series offers 18 CME credits per year. The program was favorably reviewed in the March 1992 issue of *Medical Software Reviews*. Decker also publishes a similar series from the American Academy of Otolaryngology titled Patient of the Month. This series offers 32 CME credits for eight issues and costs $375. It was reviewed in the same issue of *Medical Software Reviews*.

Health Sciences Consortium

Health Sciences Consortium acts as distributor for medical education programs developed at their member institutions. They have computer-based educational material, interactive videodisks, and videotapes for medicine, dentistry, nursing, and allied health professions. Much of their medical material is written for students, but some programs may be of general interest, including a program on arterial blood gases and a series of diagnostic problem cases. One CME program, AIDS Clinical Vignettes, offers 2.5 hours of Category 1 CME credit. The subject matter is quite broad, and prices vary from $150 for diskette programs to $1300 for larger CD-ROM programs. Consortium members get a 30% discount; about two thirds of all American medical schools are members. Membership for most United States institutions costs $1000 per year; for community nonteaching hospitals, the cost is $1000 for 2 years. A catalog is available on request.

Keyboard Publishing

Keyboard Publishing distributes a number of Macintosh Hypercard programs on pharmacology, microbiology, and pathology. For a single user, these cost from $150 to $915. Most of these programs are aimed at medical students. One program, The Acid-Base Diagnostician, offers CME credit and is a multimedia approach to teaching acid-base metabolism; up to 4 hours of credit are offered. Keyboard makes extensive use of videodisk material for teaching histology, microbiology, and other visual material. They also supply the Slice of Life videodisk with its extensive library of medical images. In addition, Keyboard sells A.D.A.M., a CD-ROM product whose excellent animated atlas of human anatomy can be manipulated to simulate dissections or surgical procedures.

Mosby-Yearbook, Inc.

Mosby, in collaboration with the American College of Physicians (ACP), has created an electronic version of ACP's popular Medical Knowledge Self-Assessment Program (MKSAP). This CD-ROM product is called MKSAP 10 Electronic and includes all the text from the MKSAP 10 program, covering current clinical information in 17 disciplines of internal medicine in syllabi, bibliographies, and multiple-choice questions. MKSAP 10 Electronic uses a book metaphor to enable the user to review, browse, and search the entire MKSAP 10 contents. The electronic product enhances the browsing and review process with full-color illustrations, video clips, and animation. The full text of articles in the MKSAP 10 bibliography is also easily accessible on the MKSAP 10 Electronic CD-ROM.

The self-assessment function of MKSAP is augmented in MKSAP 10 Electronic by automatic test scoring and test interpretation. Instant feedback on the rationale for both correct and incorrect responses are provided. Continuing medical education credits are available from ACP. MKSAP 10 is available for Windows and Macintosh computers, is priced at $395 for ACP members, and will be available in fall 1995.

Scientific American Medicine

Scientific American publishes a series of patient management problems under the title DISCOTEST. These are available both on CD-ROM, packaged with the full text of their textbook at no extra charge, and on disk. The disk-based series costs $106.95 per year for subscribers to Scientific American Medicine and

$169.95 for nonsubscribers; it is available for DOS, Windows, and Macintosh computers. DISCOTEST is published four times a year and offers up to 32 hours of CME credit if all of the cases are completed.

The computer-based cases are almost identical in content and format to the paper-based version. Figure 7-1 shows examples from a DISCOTEST patient management problem. Personally, I find these cases easier to use on paper because of the large blocks of text to read. The major advantage to the computer version is getting immediate scoring and feedback rather than having to mail in an answer sheet for scoring. Additionally, with the computer, you can reuse each case as often as you wish, trying alternative pathways, something that is obviously impossible to do with the paper version.

Williams and Wilkins Electronic Media

Williams and Wilkins has the largest library of medical education software, including the RxDx series, authored at Massachusetts General Hospital in Boston. Programs in the RxDx series generally fall into one of two formats. In one series of programs, Exercises in Clinical Problem Solving, you are presented with an initial brief case description and then asked to try to arrive at a diagnosis by gathering further clinical and laboratory data from a large menu, with as much computer assistance as you wish. Programs in this format deal with abdominal pain, anemia, bleeding disorders, chest pain, pediatric cough and fever, thyroid diseases, joint pain, and stupor and coma.

The other RxDx format offers programs in the more traditional multiple-choice style, presenting material and asking you to make a choice, at which point the results of your decision are shown and you make your next decision. Programs in this format include simulations and tutorials. Titles are Advanced Problems in Cardiac Arrhythmias, Arrhythmias Case Studies, Arrhythmias Tutorials, Arterial Blood Gases, Basic Life Support, CPR Training by Computer (BLS/ACLS), Diagnosis and Management of Acute Myocardial Infarction, Hyperlipidemia, Hypertensive Emergencies, and Management of Chronic Hypertension. These programs are sold to individual users for $98.50 and on an institutional multiuser basis for $345. CME credits of 3 to 6 hours, depending on the program, are available through Harvard Medical School.

Williams and Wilkins also publishes three programs in a series developed by the George Washington University Medical Center called Clinical Problems in Emergency Medicine: Acute Respiratory Distress, the Alcoholic Patient, and the Unresponsive Patient. These are priced at $94.50 and awarded 4 CME credits. The Unresponsive Patient was favorably reviewed in the November 1994 issue of *Medical Software Reviews*.

CD-ROM Products for Continuing Medical Education

As discussed earlier, the relatively small amount of educational material on CD-ROM can be expected to expand rapidly in the near future.

Figure 7-1. Examples of a patient management problem from DISCOTEST. Top, left. Beginning of a case presentation. **Top, right.** Split screen shows additional patient information and the physician's management options at this point in the case. **Bottom, left.** Feedback to physician on overall performance. **Bottom, right.** Scoring for different management decisions.

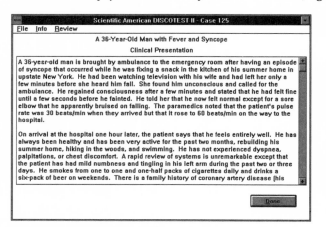

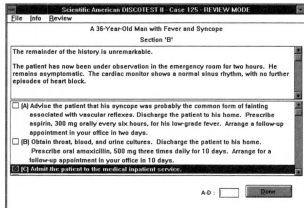

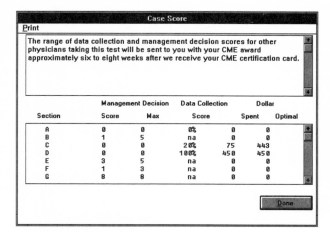

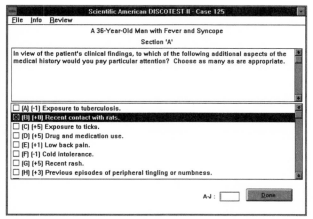

BDR, Inc.

UpToDate in Nephrology and Hypertension is a CD-ROM–based resource that readily provides answers to common diagnostic and therapeutic questions in 500 topic areas. For each question relating to therapy, a specific recommendation is made. All information, including therapy recommendations, is fully referenced. In most cases, the MEDLINE reference can be displayed with the click of a mouse.

The disc is updated every 4 months. The information in UpToDate is written by a team of internationally recognized clinicians and teachers. Complementing the text are full-color and gray-scale images, including graphs, renal histology, radiographs, and urine sediment abnormalities. A subset of MEDLINE citations is also available on the disc. UpToDate products in other medical specialty areas are under development, and questions and answers in these areas are available for preview on the Nephrology and Hypertension disc at no extra charge. The text-only version of UpToDate is being made available for the Newton personal digital assistant (PDA) (see Chapter 10).

As an accredited CME sponsor, the AMA has designated using UpToDate as a CME activity for which the user may receive one Category 1 CME credit for each hour of use. UpToDate automatically maintains a log of the date, time of day, question screen(s) reviewed, and the length of time each answer is reviewed. Users can then print the log and send it to BDR, Inc., which will obtain the AMA Category 1 CME certificate for the user for an annual fee of $50.

Continuing Medical Education Associates, Inc.

CMEA has a medical CD-ROM catalog that offers a number of products, including textbooks and journals on CD-ROM. Two journals, Mayo Clinic Proceedings and Family Practice Recertification, offer CME credits at no additional cost. Both sell for $295. The Mayo Clinic Proceedings, 1991 to 1993, offers 20 hours of CME credit; Family Practice Recertification, December 1989 to December 1993, offers 40 hours. Another available title on CD-ROM is Clinical Dermatology Illustrated, priced at $199 and offering 20 CME credit hours.

HealthCare Information Services, Inc.

HealthCare Information Services has begun offering self-assessment products in conjunction with its BiblioMed series of medical reference sources on CD-ROM. The BiblioMed Gastroenterology CD-ROM, sponsored by the American College of Gastroenterology (ACG), includes a gastroenterology-focused set of MEDLINE abstracts since 1989; the full text of the *American Journal of Gastroenterology* (including illustrations and tables) from 1992; the full text of the past 5 years from *The New England Journal of Medicine;* references and illustrations from the ACG board review courses; and an ACG self-assessment examination. The latter contains high-resolution color and black-and-white photographs (including radiographs), provides instant feedback and explains answers, and offers 12 credits upon successful completion. This disc costs $225 per year for one annual update and can be purchased along with the references Physicians GenRx or Liver and Biliary Diseases (edited by Neil Kaplowitz, MD, and published by Williams and Wilkins) for an additional $95 each.

IVI Publishing

PrimePractice, a quarterly CD-ROM CME program produced with the Mayo Clinic by IVI Publishing, is a visually and intellectually appealing product. Each quarterly disc focuses on a single specialty: The first four are scheduled to be cardiology, neurology, hypertension, and pulmonary medicine. PrimePractice uses actual heart sounds, x-rays, and so on in its case presentations. The charter subscription rate is $495 per year or $1295 for 3 years. This program offers up to 40 CME credits per year.

Reuters Health Information Services, Inc.

GeoMedica, a product of Reuters Health Information Services is a comprehensive information, communication, and education service for physicians. GeoMedica offers specialty-specific, monthly CME titles on CD-ROM. Demonstrations of diagnostic tests, medical procedures, and lectures by leading authorities are accompanied by schematic diagrams and printed text of the video segments. GeoMedica allows you to earn AMA/PRA Category 1 and Category 2 credits. Figure 7-2 shows examples of computer screens from GeoMedica's CME component.

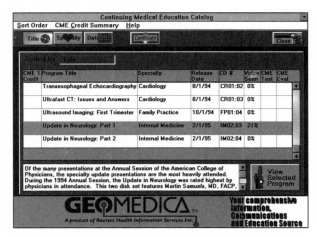
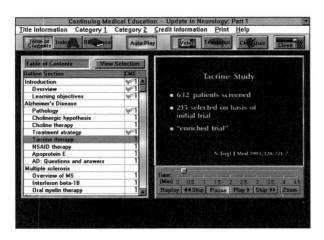

Figure 7-2. GeoMedica screens. Left. Screen shows a partial index of CME programs, with Update in Neurology: Part 1 highlighted. **Right.** Screen shows a slide presented in the Update in Neurology: Part 1 program on the right and the program's table of contents on the left.

SilverPlatter Education, Inc.

SilverPlatter offers several multimedia CME products in its collection of Multimedia Accelerated Learning offerings. These programs include the Core Curriculum in Primary Care Series, which currently consists of nine CD-ROM disks that contain several hours of lecture material, slides, and handouts from a primary care lecture series offered by several medical schools in Boston. Users can obtain up to 4 hours of AMA Category 1 credit for each disk. The Diagnostic Challenge Series uses multimedia to present users with clinical cases, provides interactive "physician tools" that enable users to make diagnostic and treatment decisions, and then compares your management to that of an expert. The first case has been released, offers CME credit, and costs $99. A third type of CME offering provides in-depth, multimedia coverage (for example, includes radiologic studies) of specific topics, as on the Etiology of Cancer disc, and enables the user to earn CME credits. The AMA is the accredited sponsor for SilverPlatter's CME programs.

HOW CAN I SUCCESSFULLY IMPLEMENT COMPUTER-BASED CME?

What Kind of Computer Do I Need?

No matter what IBM-compatible or Macintosh computer you use, you can find CME software that runs on it. If you are in the planning-to-purchase stage and CME programs are part of your planned use, you would be wise to include a CD-ROM player in your computer configuration. Although CD-ROM products are still in the minority, their advantages for educational software are so obvious that their use will certainly mushroom. Purchasing the hardware will also enable you to begin building an electronic reference library (*see* Chapter 9). Multimedia programs may require special software and hardware for you to display audio and full-motion video. You should check the requirements for programs of interest and make sure your computer configuration is appropriate.

How Do I Select Appropriate Programs?

How can you select software that is useful? Short of getting the material with the opportunity to return it—which publishers may be reluctant to do since it is so easy to copy—you are advised to seek published reviews of programs you are considering buying. Some software publishers may provide a demonstration disk, which is noted in individual advertisement descriptions. (*See* the Introduction to this book for further discussion of selecting useful software.)

A Word about Prices

Most general-purpose software has a list price and a "street price," the price you expect to pay at a discount store. Given the much smaller market for medical software, getting a bargain is not as easy, but it is worth looking. One potential source for CME (and other) software at a discount is the distributor Alpha Media. For members, the AMA is another source. In the AMA's Spring 1994 catalog, the Williams and

Wilkins program titled CPR Training by Computer was listed with a member price of $78.80, compared with the nonmember price of $98.50. The AMA also sells a number of CD-ROM products below list price. Similarly, the American College of Physicians offers medical software to members at a discount in its product catalog.

Keeping Track of CME Credits

Even if you never use a computer-based educational program, the computer can be helpful in keeping records of your CME activities. Many states and specialty societies now require you to accumulate a specified minimum number of credit hours in specific areas. On demand, you must be able to document these credits. While many of us doubtless follow the "shoebox method" of tracking CME credits, spreadsheet programs can help you organize your record keeping. There is also a shareware program, written by Robert A. Fuld, MD, that keeps track of CME credits and can be downloaded from MedSIG (Medical Special Interest Group) on CompuServe (see Chapter 8).

Incorporating Computer-based CME into a Practice: One Scenario

Although everyone develops a unique CME system based on individual needs and interests, the following case study might help you picture a successful approach to computer-based CME.

Dr. Jones is a general internist in solo practice in a mid-sized town. Her state board requires 50 hours of Category 1 CME credits annually. While she tries to get to one comprehensive postgraduate course a year, and her local hospital sponsors a monthly university-run Grand Rounds, she always finds herself scrambling to get enough credits. Many of the hospital's educational programs, which she attends primarily for the credits, do not focus on the issues she would most like to pursue.

Dr. Jones (also a closet adventure-novel writer) has an IBM-compatible 486 computer at home for writing her novels and tracking family finances. She also recently bought an IBM-compatible portable computer for writing on the go. Frustrated with her inability to conveniently access medical information in print form, Dr. Jones has already begun to explore computer-based medical information resources. During this exploration, she became acquainted with several computer-based CME products and was excited about their potential for helping her obtain accessible CME and required credits.

After reading reviews of several available products in the American College of Physicians' *Software for Internists* and talking to some computer-using colleagues, Dr. Jones purchased several floppy-disk–based programs and worked through them. While they were not awe-inspiring for the most part—being of the traditional, simple, multiple-choice format—Dr. Jones found the programs interesting, informative, and convenient for accumulating the needed CME credits. She generally uses the programs for a few hours each month in the evenings or on rainy weekend days. Increasingly, she has been using them on her portable computer during free time in her busy week. Recently, she purchased a computer program for tracking her CME credits and is pleased that she no longer has to face the unpleasant task of trying to reconstruct such a log, hoping that the total hours will add up to at least the "magic number."

Recognizing the power of CD-ROM technology for delivering massive amounts of text (as well as pictures, sounds, and video), Dr. Jones is planning to buy a CD-ROM player for her home computer to access both medical resources for herself and encyclopedic resources for her family. She is planning to purchase at least one medical CD-ROM program that combines information resources with CME offerings. She also has her eye on upgrading her computer at home to take advantage of the new generation of multimedia CME programs now visible on the horizon.

Dr. Jones has found that computer-based CME, while not yet a magic bullet for overcoming all of CME's difficulties, is a cost-effective, useful, and enjoyable resource for meeting this important professional obligation. She excitedly anticipates the further growth and maturation of these products.

8

TELECOMMUNICATIONS

Paul Kleeberg, MD; and Daniel R. Masys, MD, FACP

HOW CAN COMPUTER TELECOMMUNICATIONS HELP ME IN MY PRACTICE?

The power and information storage capacity of the modern personal computer are quite remarkable, but the computer's full potential is realized only when one takes advantage of its ability to communicate with other information sources, systems, and computer users. Your machine can be a window on the world, capable of exploring and bringing back information from thousands of miles away with no more difficulty than it manages information stored on its own disk.

Telecommunications can enhance your medical practice in many ways, giving you the potential to do the following:

- Get a concise, up-to-date synopsis of disease treatment (for a newly diagnosed cancer patient,

for example, treatment information [and a patient-education printout] is obtainable from the online database of the National Cancer Institute's PDQ [Physician Data Query])

- Gain instant access to a patient's records from any location equipped with similar telecommunications capabilities

- Get laboratory test results at your home computer by connecting to your hospital's laboratory information system when you are covering over the weekend

- Send and receive medical images (for example, electrocardiograms, magnetic resonance imaging scans, x-rays), which can be viewed on your computer screen

- Read and post notes to electronic bulletin boards read by hundreds or even thousands of other persons with similar interests, ranging from medical subspecialties to travel, hobbies, and finance

- Communicate via electronic mail (e-mail) with colleagues and friends, including those who reside in different states or even different countries
- Download new software programs, including demonstration versions of medical software, or run medical programs that are resident on other machines (for example, run QMR from Physicians' Online)
- Search the medical literature and other databases from the National Library of Medicine (NLM) and other information providers.

Telecommunications at Work: Four Scenarios

The value of the different features and varied functionality of telecommunications may be experienced routinely by physicians in all aspects of practice. The scenarios that follow illustrate some of the capabilities noted above, and they incorporate some additional information that will be discussed in this chapter.

SCENARIO 1: ONLINE RESEARCH FOR TREATMENT RECOMMENDATIONS. A 21-year-old patient presents to your office with the diagnosis of Friedreich ataxia. Luckily, he already knows his diagnosis, but he also knows he feels lousy and wants to feel better. That is your job. A quick check through your texts in the office yields little helpful information. Additionally, some of your books are not recent editions, so you are not sure if there is more current information. A MEDLINE search would give references to the current literature, but you are not sure if that would help you manage this patient. A search of Victor McKusick's *Online Mendelian Inheritance in Man* does yield a succinct description of Friedreich ataxia along with inheritance patterns, treatment recommendations, and references.

SCENARIO 2: PROVIDING PATIENT EDUCATION VIA THE PDQ DATABASE. A man who had Wilms tumor as a child wants to know what the likelihood is of passing the disease on to his children. Again, you could look in the books in your office for information, but given the recent advances in genetic research, you are not confident that the material is accurate. Searching the PDQ database using CompuServe shows that the likelihood of your patient's passing his condition on to his offspring is less than 2%, since he had unilateral disease.

SCENARIO 3: STAYING CONNECTED THROUGH E-MAIL. A physician who lives in rural Minnesota has a special interest in the use of information technology in medical practice. She has been to several medical meetings and has enjoyed seeing the new technology and listening to the lectures. Even more stimulating were the conversations she had with the people she met there. She knew from experience with previous conferences that despite plans to keep in touch, these connections usually ended with the plane flight home. This time she vowed it would be different. She copied down the e-mail address of everyone she met there who was interested in information technology in rural practice. After returning home, she sent out an e-mail message to the entire group, listing all names and addresses. Later, when she read an article about a physician in California who was proposing to treat patients using two-way interactive multimedia in their homes without the benefit of a local caregiver, she reproduced it for the group and sent it out. She enjoyed "listening in" to the heated discussion that ensued and discovered that she could learn a great deal from the more vocal members as they argued their position.

SCENARIO 4: KEEPING ON TOP OF THE MEDICAL NEWS. Another physician who wishes to stay abreast of the medical news appearing in the local newspapers frequently scans the "Health and Medicine in the News" Gopher maintained by the University of Minnesota medical library (*see under* Gopher: Navigating by Menu). They have a librarian who reads the Twin Cities newspaper, scanning for medically related articles. The librarian then posts a summary of the article along with relevant references from the medical literature. The physician finds that by scanning this resource he is often able to know the details about a news release before his patients start asking him in the clinic.

WHAT TELECOMMUNICATIONS RESOURCES AND PRODUCTS ARE AVAILABLE?

There are two approaches to answering this question. One is to discuss the types of information and communication resources available online. The other is to describe individual service providers in terms of what they provide. We shall approach this issue from both perspectives.

We describe online resources that are available in six categories:

- Electronic mail
- Discussion groups
- Bulletin boards, newsgroups, and forums
- Newsletters
- Information repositories
- Internet navigation systems.

Service providers in five categories are also described:

- E-mail access providers
- Value-added services
- Bulletin board systems
- Information repository vendors
- Internet access providers.

Types of Telecommunications Resources

Electronic Mail

Electronic mail, or e-mail, is the most basic service that telecommunications provides, yet in many ways it is the most powerful. When you get an account on a networked computer system, the system administrator generally gives you a unique user name (user ID) to use along with a password to log onto the system. The computer identifies you as an authorized user from your ID. Your secret password prevents other users from logging onto the system with your ID. Your user ID–password combination allows you to maintain a private area on the computer system and also makes it possible for you to send and receive e-mail. The central computer(s) to which users are connected is generally called the "host," while the user's computer is referred to as the "local" machine. The local computer (and user) are said to be "online" while connected to the host over a network.

E-mail is nothing more than digital information sent from one user to other users. The e-mail sender or receiver(s) can be on the same host machine or on different hosts connected to each other over a network. E-mail messages may also contain attached files such as encoded images, sound, specially formatted text, or multimedia files.

The typical e-mail message contains a header with information about the date the message was sent, the sender, and the intended recipient(s), and a subject line indicating the topic of the message. Next comes the body of the message, which may include text or other information, or both, and finally a "signature," which many e-mail writers use to convey personal information such as their affiliation, telephone and fax numbers, and so forth.

E-mail gets its power from its ability to bring people together, much the same as the telephone. The advantages of e-mail are several. First, e-mail has the ability to allow for asynchronous conversation—people communicating back and forth on their own time and at their own convenience, without having to be synchronously in contact with one another (much like a telephone "conversation" where two persons talk only to the other's answering machine). With e-mail, you can also attach files to the message.

Theoretically, portions of a medical record can be transmitted this way, but issues of security and confidentiality must be considered. And e-mail enables you to send messages to more than one person at the same time. E-mail is also the most often-used method to "post" a message in a host computer's public area when you want more than one person to see it.

Most service providers allow for e-mail; and many, but not all, providers allow you to mail to individuals outside of their system. This factor is important to know when subscribing to a service, since all whom you wish to contact may not be on your host system.

Discussion Groups

Online dialogue among groups of people with similar interests is one of the most popular aspects of telecommunications. These electronic interactions have been compared to a "virtual dinner party" where you can wander from conversation to conversation, either taking an active role or just listening in. Almost any topic you can imagine is discussed online; literally thousands of discussion groups are on the Internet, each devoted to a different topic. Furthermore, the number of these discussion groups is growing rapidly.

Online discussion takes place in two basic ways. In one model, each person's contribution to the discussion is automatically e-mailed to all other participants. This type of interaction is called a discussion group, or a "listserve list," and is described below. The other method is called a bulletin board (or newsgroup or forum) and is discussed in the next section. Even though these types of online interaction are distinct, you should be aware that the names are sometimes used interchangeably.

Discussion groups are a variation of person-to-person e-mail. Someone wishing to contribute to a discussion sends an e-mail message with her or his comments to a special software program (often called a listserver) on a host computer. The listserver then automatically forwards the message to a list of e-mail addresses belonging to discussion group members, which is stored in the listserver software. To join a discussion group and receive these messages, you must send a request to the "list owner," or person responsible for the discussion group. Many discussion groups can be joined automatically by sending a specially formatted e-mail message to an administrative address for the listserver that instructs the program to add your name to the list. In either case, this process is referred to as "subscribing" to the list or discussion group. Similarly, participants can "unsubscribe." Announcements for listserve lists on a topic generally describe the purpose of the list, the address and format for requests to subscribe or unsubscribe, and the address to which you send messages for the other subscribers on the list.

At last count, over 300 medically related discussion groups were on the Internet alone. As with general-interest discussion groups, the number of medically related lists is growing rapidly. Here are a few examples:

Addiction	Cancer
Aging	Clinical alerts
AIDS	Cystic fibrosis
Autism	Diabetes

Emergency medicine	Medical students
Fitness	Multiple sclerosis
Health management	Nursing homes
Health reform	Parkinson disease
Hospital news	Schizophrenia
Immunizations	Stroke
Lyme disease	Student health
Medical librarians	Women's health

Discussion groups can be an enjoyable and educational opportunity to participate in a discussion on a topic of interest to you. The other participants can be from anywhere on the globe, so the discussion group can help to expand your perspective. You have the opportunity to formulate your thoughts without being interrupted; and when your ideas are challenged, you have the opportunity to develop your thoughts further. Discussion groups are ideal for continuing a conversation after a conference when the participants have returned home.

Remember that discussion groups distribute their messages as e-mail, which is an advantage if you wish to receive mailings from a list in which postings are infrequent. Postings appear in your "electronic inbox," which you can check whenever you log onto your host computer. Thus, with discussion groups, you do not have to remember to check regularly a location other than your e-mail inbox.

Additionally, many discussion groups require membership for posting, and some groups are "moderated." List owners of moderated groups screen the posts before they are distributed to the subscribers. Some groups require membership to post a message to prevent inappropriate or mistaken postings.

Discussion groups are not without problems. New users often sign up for several discussion groups and soon find that they have trouble keeping up with their mail. When a particular discussion gets heated, the messages can become frequent and lengthy, causing your e-mail inbox to overflow. And messages continue to be stored in your inbox while you are away on vacation, which can cause more important messages to get lost if your inbox fills while you are gone.

Bulletin Boards, Newsgroups, and Forums

These resources are similar to discussion groups with one significant difference. Rather than distribute the messages as mail in your inbox, the bulletin board (or newsgroup or forum) saves the messages in a common area in which anyone with access to the host system where the bulletin board resides may browse. An analogy is the (nonelectronic) bulletin board near many hospital cafeterias. There are hundreds of newsgroups on the Internet and forums on CompuServe, America Online, and many other vendors. Unlike discussion groups for which you "sign up" to participate, you can merely "drop in" to an area to read its bulletin board or newsgroup messages. Currently, many online services are actively cultivating medically related forums.

One advantage of the newsgroup-forum format compared with discussion groups is that they do not clog your mailbox. Following a "thread" (that is, a series of messages on a particular topic from within a newsgroup) is also easier because the messages within a newsgroup and forum are arranged according to subject.

Disadvantages of some newsgroups and forums are that the membership may be more transient, providing less of a sense of community among the users. (Many discussion groups require membership for posting, so transience is less of a problem for them.) Some forums, for example, the American College of Physicians' (ACP) forum ACP Online on CompuServe, limit access to a certain group of people (ACP members for ACP Online), narrowing the focus of the newsgroup. MedSIG, a popular medically oriented forum open to all subscribers and sponsored by the American Medical Informatics Association (AMIA), is also available on CompuServe.

Newsletters

Several medically oriented newsletters are available online. Just as with postings to discussion groups, these newsletters appear in your electronic mailbox at regular intervals. Some of these also appear in print, but many do not. *AIDS Daily Summary* is a clipping service from the Centers for Disease Control and Prevention, and it is very popular. *Health Info-Com Newsletter* is a biweekly newsletter that contains clippings from *U.S. News and World Report,* an electronic copy of the *Morbidity and Mortality Weekly Report,* software reviews, conference announcements, and feature articles.

Information Repositories

Three types of information repositories accessible online are databases, decision support systems, and software archives.

DATABASES. Using an online database is often the best way to get the most current information. Several text and bibliographic databases are searchable online. The most well-known medical bibliographic database is MEDLINE, maintained by the NLM. Full-text databases include the PDQ Cancernet database and *Online Mendelian Inheritance in Man,* among many others. You can browse these centrally located archives of information using a keyword search. *(See* Chapters 3 and 9 for more detailed discussions on bibliographic and text databases.)

DECISION SUPPORT SYSTEMS. Some vendors (for example, Physicians' Online and US HealthLink) provide online access to decision support systems such as QMR and DXplain (*see* Chapter 4). These systems analyze signs, symptoms, and laboratory results to generate a differential diagnosis based on the information you provide. Some of these systems suggest additional tests to do to help in diagnosis.

SOFTWARE ARCHIVES. Most commercial vendors and many Internet sites have software archives, which are areas containing software that you can retrieve and use on your personal computer. Some of these programs are "freeware" (you may use it for free), and some are "shareware" (try it, and if you wish to keep it, you send the author a modest registration fee). Many software vendors also distribute demonstration versions of their software and version updates in these archives. Several medically oriented software archives are available on the Internet, including sites maintained by the University of Texas Medical School; the University of California, Irvine; and the State University of Campanas, Brazil. Selected demonstration versions of medically

related software are available on ACP Online and on MedSIG.

Internet Navigation Systems

Before we talk about navigating the Internet, a word or two about the network itself. The Internet is a loosely connected network of networks, international in scope, linking several million computers in dozens of countries around the world. The Internet grew out of computer communications standards developed by the U.S. Defense Department in the 1970s and was primarily a communications network linking colleges, universities, and computer centers until the late 1980s. Now the restrictions on access to the Internet are being lifted, and many commercial companies have host computers on the network; virtually all of the commercial online vendors can forward and receive e-mail to the Internet computers (and thereby to each other).

The principal benefits of the Internet lie in the speed with which it processes communications and in the volume of people it can serve. The Internet provides communications speeds which are 10 to 100 times faster than those available over telephone lines via modem; this makes it practical to send very large files, for example, those required to transmit color images, sound, and even motion pictures. In addition, vast numbers of computer users can simultaneously send mail to, and participate within, electronic bulletin board "conferences" or informal information exchanges. Many of the host computers on the Internet have public file areas that allow anyone to read and retrieve their files. Some information service providers, such as the NLM, make special multimedia "hypertext" documents such as text and color graphics of clinical practice guidelines available via the Internet.

But locating the Internet resources that interest you is not necessarily a simple or straightforward matter. In fact, navigating the Internet can be downright difficult, although this challenge is characterized in widely different terms according to who describes it.

Several different interface systems enable users to navigate the Internet—that is, to access documents and computers around the world that are connected to the Internet. In order to become a part of this grand network—which is in fact a tangled web of computers of different brands and different operating systems—the would-be participating machines have to agree on only a few basic principles: how to exchange mail, how to exchange files, and how to allow someone from another system to log on. In computer parlance, a set of agreed-upon rules shared by communicating systems is called a protocol. Tools such as FTP, which stands for file transfer protocol, enable users to retrieve files from other computers on the Internet; a utility called TELNET enables users to actually log onto these remote computers.

Enter Gopher and Mosaic: These two popular and useful interfaces to FTP, TELNET, and other powerful Internet utilities can help you access medical information on the Internet.

Gopher: Navigating by Menu

Gopher is a program designed to simplify the task of navigating the Internet. It shows a menu of functions you can access on the network. Created in 1991, Gopher provided an easy menu-based interface for retrieving documents from computer systems scattered around the world. Before 1991, the only way to retrieve a file on the Internet was by knowing both the name of the machine where the file was located and the path to the subdirectory in which the file resided. In those pre-Gopher days, "surfing the Internet" in search of useful information was not for the faint of heart. More important, it was very difficult to find anything.

Gopher created a menu-driven interface to these resources. It freed the user from having to learn complex commands, and it made browsing through the Internet much easier. The client-server architecture of Gopher automatically took care of passing these archaic commands between the client (or local) and server (or host) systems. Files could be searched and application programs retrieved merely by selecting items from a menu.

Predominantly an Internet tool, Gopher has become so popular that it is quickly spreading to the commercial online vendors as well. In fact, many commercial vendors are beginning to provide access to the Internet Gopher because the resources on the Internet far outstrip anything they could provide alone.

The medical practitioner can find great benefit here. Some examples of the many resources available through the Gopher databases are:

- PDQ database and Online Mendelian Inheritance in Man (both of which can be searched using keywords)

- Back issues of the electronic newsletters

- Computers at the NLM, National Institutes of Health (NIH), National Cancer Institute, the

White House, Johns Hopkins, and Stanford (as well as many other universities)

- Medical-software archives and discussion-group archives.

This list is just a small sampling of the Internet resources made readily accessible through Gopher. In June 1993, there were 1300 Gopher servers—computers that allowed one to search their files with Gopher. By October 1994, that number had grown to 4809.

Mosaic: Multimedia and More

Mosaic is an exemplar of a new generation of graphical interfaces to the Internet. First developed for UNIX workstations, versions of this software were released for the Macintosh and for PCs running Windows in late 1993. Much like Gopher, Mosaic enabled a point-and-click interface to computer systems around the world, but it took things one important step further. Instead of only being able to view unformatted text documents on your screen, authors were now able to deliver documents with text formatting (for example, italics, underline, bold, font changes) as well as color images, sounds, and movies to many other personal computers around the world. And users were enabled to access this material via a user-friendly interface. Documents could appear, formatted just as on the printed page; however, words or icons within those documents could be linked to other files, text strings, still images, movies, or sounds anywhere on the network. Suddenly, the electronic page itself came alive at the same time that it integrated information from computers around the

world. For example, through links to resources such as the Virtual Hospital:

- The cough of a child with croup can be heard with the click of a mouse on a highlighted area in a document
- The ataxic gait of a person with Parkinson disease can be watched in action
- The chest x-ray of a patient with a small pneumothorax can be retrieved and viewed from a remote computer for teaching purposes.

Mosaic was developed by the National Center for Supercomputing Applications (NCSA) and can be downloaded free of charge from the NCSA computers. Commercial software that performs similar functions is becoming available. Netscape, available free to end users, is a popular example.

Mosaic and similar software have two main disadvantages. First, it requires either a direct link to the Internet or a special dial-up connection (Serial Line Internet Protocol [SLIP] or Point to Point Protocol [PPP]; *see under* Connecting to Internet via Modem). These are available at many academic centers and through several commercial vendors (*see under* Types of Providers of Online Services), but they are not yet ubiquitous. Second, sound and image files are hundreds of times larger than text files, and full-motion video files can be hundreds of times larger than sound and image files. The result is that transferring these documents is slow and requires faster modems, faster personal computers (for interpreting the images, sounds, and so on), and larger storage capacity, both in memory and on the hard drive.

Types of Providers of Online Services

From e-mail to discussion groups, bulletin boards, newsletters, clinical information sources, and the vast Internet, the array of telecommunications resources is there, ready to be explored. How do you get to these resources? You get there through the various providers of online services. As described earlier, there are different kinds of telecommunications service providers; they roughly correspond to the resource categories we have described and may be organized under five main headings: 1) e-mail access providers; 2) value-added services; 3) bulletin board systems; 4) information repository vendors; and 5) Internet access providers. The individual service providers discussed here are listed in Table 8-1.

E-mail Access Providers

Some online services provide you with e-mail access only. For individuals without any other mode of access to online systems for e-mail exchange, this type of service is a great place to start. Providers generally give you a user ID, password, software to connect to the system, and a toll-free number to use to send and retrieve mail.

AT&T EASYLINK SERVICES. This service features a low, flat monthly fee with toll-free dial-in access. You pay to send mail and for connect time. Receiving mail is free. The service has no software for downloading or interest groups. AT&T Easylink enables you to send e-mail to anyone on the Internet or on another network connected to the Internet via a gateway.

MCI MAIL. This service features a low yearly fee with toll-free dial-in access. You pay to send mail. Receiving mail and online time is free. MCI Mail is useful as an e-mail address for rural physicians and others who want to use e-mail but are a long-distance call from any of the value-added services described below. No software for downloading or interest groups is available. Like the above service, MCI Mail enables you to send e-mail to anyone on the Internet or on another network connected to the Internet via a gateway.

SPRINTMAIL. This service is more expensive than the other two. You pay to send mail, receive mail, and for connect time. The service is business-oriented and has no software for downloading or interest groups. Like the two other services, SprintMail enables you to send e-mail to anyone on the Internet or on another network connected to the Internet via a gateway.

Value-Added Services

Most of the online service providers fall within this category. These value-added providers are basically dedicated "host" computers that the vendor loads with useful information and communication services. Using a modem, users access the host computer by dialing into local numbers on national communication networks such as CompuServe, Sprintnet, or Tymnet. (Note that CompuServe provides nationwide network access as well as the separate value-added service described below.)

Value-added services provide e-mail along with forums, shareware and freeware that you can download, and text archives. Several of these vendors provide useful nonmedical services and databases such as stock quotes, weather forecasts from around the country, airline ticket ordering and information, movie and consumer product reviews, and much

Table 8-1. Online Services and Providers

Online Service and Providers	Address of Provider	Phone and Fax Numbers, E-mail Address of Provider	
E-mail access			
AT&T EasyLink Services	Room 1015 5501 LBJ Freeway Dallas, TX 75240	Tel: Fax:	800-242-6005 214-778-5024 214-778-4235
MCI Mail	1133 19th Street, N.W. Seventh Floor Washington, DC 20036	Tel: Fax:	800-444-6245 202-736-6000 800-677-3303
SprintMail	1200 Main Street Fourth Floor Kansas City, MO 64105	Tel: Fax:	800-736-1130 800-359-4011
Value-added services			
America Online	8619 Westwood Center Drive Vienna, VA 22182	Tel: Fax:	800-827-6364 703-883-1509
BIX	1030 Massachusetts Avenue Cambridge, MA 02138	Tel: Fax:	800-695-4775 617-441-4903
CompuServe	5000 Arlington Centre Boulevard P.O. Box 20212 Columbus, OH 43220	Tel: Fax:	800-848-8199 614-457-8600 614-457-0348
Delphi Internet Services Corp.	1030 Massachusetts Avenue Cambridge, MA 02138	Tel: Fax: E-mail:	800-695-4005 617-491-3393 617-441-4903 info@delphi.com
GEnie	401 North Washington Street Rockville, MD 20850	Tel: Fax: E-mail:	800-638-9636 301-251-6421 feedback@genie. geis.com
Physicians' Online	560 White Plains Road Tarrytown, NY 10591	Tel: Fax: E-mail:	800-332-0009 914-332-6100 914-332-6445 jsacks@po.com
Prodigy	445 Hamilton Avenue White Plains, NY 10601	Tel:	800-PRODIGY
US HealthLink	4676 Admiralty Way, #217 Marina del Rey, CA 90292	Tel: Fax:	800-682-8770 310-577-0420 310-577-0402

* The telephone number is for the modem connection to the bulletin board.

(Continued on next page)

Table 8-1. *(Continued)*

Online Service and Providers	Address of Provider	Phone and Fax Numbers, E-mail Address of Provider
Bulletin board systems		
AIDS Ministries		Tel: 800-542-5921*
Black Bag BBS		Tel: 610-454-7396* E-mail: ed@blackbag.com
FDA Bulletin Board		Tel: 800-222-0185*
FDA Medwatch Reporting		Tel: 800-332-7737*
GRATEFUL MED Support		Tel: 800-525-5756*
HNS HIV Net		Tel: 800-788-4118*
Information repositories		
CDP Technologies	333 Seventh Avenue New York, NY 10001	Tel: 800-950-2035 Fax: 212-563-3784
Knight-Ridder Information, Inc.	2440 El Camino Real Mountain View, CA 94040	Tel: 800-3-DIALOG 415-254-7000 Fax: 415-254-7070
Mead Data Central	3445 Newmark Drive Miamisburg, OH 45432	Tel: 800-227-4908 Fax: 800-348-2609
National Library of Medicine	8600 Rockville Pike Bethesda, MD 20894	Tel: 800-638-8480 Fax: 301-496-0822
PaperChase	350 Longwood Avenue Longwood Galleria Boston, MA 02115	Tel: 800-722-2075 617-278-3900 Fax: 617-277-9792
Internet access		
Colorado SuperNet, Inc.	999 Eighteenth Street Suite 2640 Denver, CO 80202	Tel: 303-296-8202 Fax: 303-296-8224
Minnesota Regional Network (MRNet)	511 11th Avenue South Box 212 Minneapolis, MN 55415	Tel: 612-342-2891 Fax: 612-342-2873 E-mail: mpalmer@mr.net
TerraNet, Inc.	729 Boylston Street Fifth Floor Boston, MA 02116	Tel: 617-450-9000 Fax: 617-450-9003

more. Except for Physicians' Online, each charges a monthly fee or for connect time, or both. In addition, many vendors charge a fee (for example, 15 cents) for sending or receiving e-mail (or for both) from the Internet. Many value-added services also provide Canadian and international access.

AMERICA ONLINE. This service provides e-mail, including a gateway which enables the exchange of e-mail with users on the Internet. Also provided are forums and software for downloading. Forums include "Ask the Doc" (oriented toward lay people) and others. Full Internet access is planned via Gopher, Mosaic, and other specialized Internet functions. Sign-up is online if you have America Online software or by dialing their business number. Access is via Sprintnet or Tymnet network numbers.

BIX. E-mail (including a gateway to Internet) and software are provided. The service also provides direct Internet access with TELNET, FTP, and Gopher. A medical forum is included. Access is via Sprintnet or Tymnet network numbers.

COMPUSERVE. This vendor provides e-mail, full Internet access, software, shareware, and forums such as MedSIG and others. MedSIG is a mature, medically oriented forum with several hundred messages posted in various different topic areas each day. A large volume of useful text and software for downloading is stored in archives called libraries.

The American College of Physicians has a private area, called ACP Online, which provides a forum where ACP members discuss medical, computing, health reform, and other topics (Figure 8-1). Clinical alerts from NIH and clinically important announcements from the Food and Drug Adminis-

tration (for example, drug recalls and new drug indications) are posted in an alerts section, as are selected clinically important announcements from ACP. In addition, libraries contain software and documents such as selected NIH consensus conferences and ACP information.

CompuServe users can search PDQ as well as access MEDLINE via the PaperChase program. Several other useful medical databases are also available. Sign-up is online if you have their software or by dialing their business number. Access is via CompuServe network numbers; Sprintnet or Tymnet access requires an additional fee.

DELPHI INTERNET SERVICES CORP. E-mail, software, and shareware are provided, as well as direct Internet access with TELNET, FTP, and Gopher. Medical forums include HealthNet, oriented primarily toward lay people, and others. Users may create their own forums. Access to Dialog Information Services is available for an additional fee. Information and sign-up are available online or by dialing the business number. Access is via Sprintnet or Tymnet network numbers.

GENIE. This service provides e-mail, Internet mail, software, and shareware. Forums include the Medical Round Table and others. Information databases are available for an additional fee. Access is via Sprintnet numbers or General Electric Information services.

PHYSICIANS' ONLINE. Through the sponsorship of pharmaceutical manufacturers, this service is free of charge to all physicians in the United States. A view of the main menu is shown in Figure 8-2 (top). Access to MEDLINE, AIDSLINE, Physicians' GenRx (Figure 8-2, bottom), and QMR is provided. Global

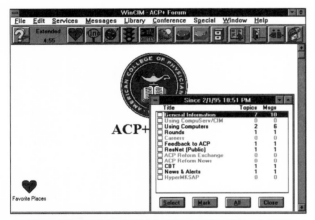

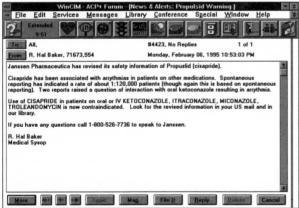

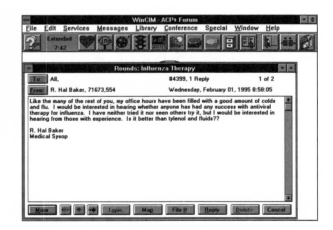

Figure 8-1. ACP Online. Top. Window showing forum message sections on top of main window. **Bottom, left.** A message regarding flu treatment is posted in the Rounds section. **Bottom, right.** A pharmaceutical warning is posted in the News & Alerts section.

e-mail and online forums are planned. Physicians' Online requires dedicated Windows or Macintosh software, which is provided free. Access is via Sprintnet or Tymnet network numbers. For rural physicians, toll-free access is under consideration.

PRODIGY. E-mail, software, and shareware are provided; an Internet mail gateway recently became operational. Several forums on health-related topics oriented primarily toward lay people are available. Databases such as Dow Jones are available for an additional fee. Access is via Sprintnet or Tymnet network numbers.

US HEALTHLINK. This service is physician oriented, providing e-mail, medical news, and bulletin boards. An Internet mail gateway is planned. Databases include MEDLINE, Disease Synopsis

Information, and Empires. Some other services include DXplain (a diagnostic decision support program), a searchable continuing medical education (CME) database, and CME patient simulations. Access is via CompuServe network numbers. This service is currently owned by Alpha Media.

Bulletin Board Systems

These systems are much like the commercial value-added services in that they provide access to e-mail, forums, and software archives, but they differ in two key aspects. First, these systems do not provide local dial-in access; in order to connect to them, one usually must call long distance. Second, these systems seldom exchange e-mail with other bulletin board systems. The following bulletin boards focus on medicine, and some of them provide toll-free access.

AIDS MINISTRIES AND HNS HIV NET. Both of these bulletin boards discuss issues such as treatment methods for HIV and AIDS patients. Users include physicians, allied health workers, and patients.

BLACK BAG BBS. This rich and mature medical bulletin board provides access to over 500 medical discussion groups from Internet and elsewhere. It contains a vast library of medical shareware programs totaling over 1 Gb and provides an online disease and symptom database along with continually updated health news, a health newsletter, *Morbidity and Mortality Weekly Report,* and more. Also available is the Black Bag Medical BBS list, which contains

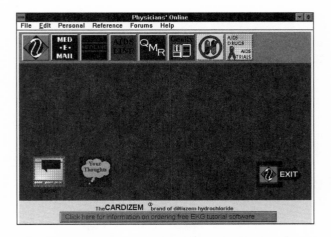

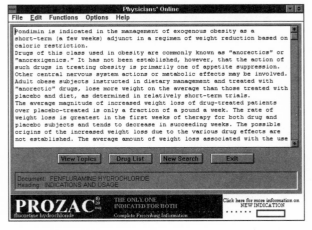

Figure 8-2. Physicians' Online. Top. Screen shows the main program options; note advertising below. **Bottom.** Extract of drug information text from Physicians' GenRx program.

pointers to over 400 online medical resources whose existence has been verified. This system requires a long-distance telephone call to connect to the BBS, but an offline reader is available.

FDA BULLETIN BOARD. Topics include news releases, enforcement reports, drug and device approvals, text from the *Drug Bulletin,* current information on AIDS, text of speeches, and important alerts. Information appears online the day it is released, and users may search the database by keywords. Access is either through remote log-in on the Internet or by dialing direct. There is no charge to the user.

FDA MEDWATCH REPORTING. This bulletin board allows health care professionals to report problems with medications and medical devices.

GRATEFUL MED SUPPORT. This service offers technical support for the users of GRATEFUL MED, a computer program that provides access to NLM's MEDLINE database.

Information Repository Vendors

These vendors are predominantly in the business of selling you information, along with some e-mail and bulletin board services.

CDP TECHNOLOGIES. CDP Colleague, formerly BRS Colleague, is a component of CDP Technologies' new online service, CDP Online. CDP Colleague is geared toward anyone requiring access to important biomedical information. Completely menu-driven, CDP Colleague provides searchable access to over 60 biomedical databases (such as MEDLINE, CancerLit, EMBASE Drug Information, Current Contents, and more) plus full-text access to 80 medical journals and 40 medical texts including the *Journal of the American Medical Association, British Medical Journal, The New*

England Journal of Medicine, The Yearbook of Medicine, and *The Yearbook of Surgery.* Online access is available through Sprintnet, Tymnet, Datapac, and the Internet.

KNIGHT-RIDDER INFORMATION, INC. With 400-plus databases, Dialog is the largest commercial collection of online databases. Dialog's "Medical Connection" databases include MEDLINE, CancerLit, drug information, and others. Full-text retrieval of 11 medical journals is offered. E-mail is available with other Dialog users only. Bulletin boards are also available. Access is via Dialnet, Sprintnet, and Tymnet network numbers. Access is also available from the Internet, reducing connect-time charges.

MEAD DATA CENTRAL. MEDIS is the medical information component of Mead Data Central's LEXIS and NEXIS online information services. There are no e-mail or bulletin board services. Databases include Updated and Archived Journals, Drug Information, FDC Reports, PDQ, MEDLINE, and Micromedex Information. The full text of 40 journals is offered. Access is via Meadnet, Sprintnet, and Tymnet network numbers.

NATIONAL LIBRARY OF MEDICINE. NLM builds and maintains MEDLINE and more than 40 other medical databases, which include HSTAT (it contains the full text of clinical practice guidelines from the Agency for Health Care Policy and Research) and PDQ (information on diagnosis and treatment in medical oncology, developed and updated by the National Cancer Institute and distributed by NLM). All databases are searchable through a command-line interface (nonfriendly but powerful), and many are searchable via GRATEFUL MED, a more user-friendly interface that helps to minimize costs by allowing the user to formulate a search offline. The software automatically connects to the NLM (either by dial-in or TELNET), logs in, searches, retrieves the results, disconnects, and saves the results for inspection offline. Both PC and Mac versions now include the Loansome Doc program, which facilitates the fax or U.S. Mail retrieval of articles selected by the searcher. Access is via Sprintnet or Tymnet. Toll-free access is available for users at remote sites, and Internet access has recently been added. Some medical societies (including ACP) provide their members with GRATE-FUL MED software and unlimited MEDLINE and other database searching time for a flat yearly fee.

PAPERCHASE. This is a menu-driven interface for MEDLINE, Health Planning and Administration, CancerLit, and AIDSLINE databases. It is also available on CompuServe. No e-mail is provided. Access is by Sprintnet or Tymnet network numbers and from the Internet.

Internet Access Providers

These services are mainly in the business of providing Internet access. They provide few resources of their own but are popular because they enable the subscriber to connect to the world of resources formerly available only to those with academic or research accounts. These providers can often help you get connected and supply you with the software necessary to get started.

Below are examples of three commercial services that provide Internet access only. They charge for initial set-up and connect time. A more complete list is contained in the document "The Public Dialup Internet Access List." To obtain this document, send an e-mail message to "info-deli-server@netcom.com"; in the body of the message, write "Send PDIAL." Of

note, Oregon Health Sciences University offers all Oregon physicians free dial-in Internet accounts that provide e-mail and access to MEDLINE.

COLORADO SUPERNET, INC. This provides SLIP access to the Internet (*see under* Connecting with Internet via Modem). A toll-free dial-in is available at a reasonable rate. Software for your computer may be provided.

MINNESOTA REGIONAL NETWORK (MRNET). This also provides SLIP access to the Internet. Software for your Mac or PC is included in sign-up charges, and a copy of *The Whole Internet User's Guide and Catalog* by Ed Krol is also included.

TERRANET, INC. This provides both SLIP and PPP access to the Internet (*see under* Connecting with Internet via Modem). Very high-speed direct connections are also available. Software for your computer may be provided.

HOW CAN I SUCCESSFULLY IMPLEMENT TELECOMMUNICATIONS TECHNOLOGY IN MY PRACTICE?

The most critical element of a successful journey into the world of telecommunications is a realistic expectation. While useful information and dialogue is certainly available now, learning when and how to access these resources successfully takes time, patience, and experience. One of the easiest ways to get started is to choose one of the commercial value-added services; pick one whose offerings seem interesting and contact them for additional information and help. Most of them provide dedicated software for their service, which makes getting started easy. Basic functions such as e-mail and forums are generally straightforward to use; user support tends to be good; some medically oriented databases or forums, or both, are available; and useful nonmedical discussions or forums, or both, are provided. Dedicated software for these vendors is also often included when you purchase a modem.

An alternative strategy would be to try Physicians' Online. This service provides customized software to connect to their system, which is free for physicians. However, you should keep in mind that Physicians' Online is not a mature service like the others, and users could experience the difficulties inherent in new software systems.

For those of you affiliated with an academic institution, you may wish to consider contacting your network services department about getting an e-mail account. Many of these accounts are provided free and can be accessed from any computer with a modem. If you are interested in searching the medical literature, the GRATEFUL MED program developed by NLM for PCs and Macintoshes (see Chapter 3) is a mature, inexpensive, and practical tool for getting started in telecommunications.

Since the idea of an "information superhighway" has captured the public imagination, the shelves of local bookstores are overflowing with how-to books for access to online information services. Popular volumes include *Internet for Dummies* and Ed Krol's *The Whole Internet*. Recent copies of PC and Macintosh magazines also contain articles about many of the commercial information services and the Internet and describe how to get started. A recent issue of *PC Computing* (September 1994) contains a lengthy, special report titled "Going I-Way?" about the Internet and other online services. Another helpful article for Macintosh users is "Plug In to the Internet" in *MacUser* (September 1994). (*See* the Appendix to this book for further reading.)

Getting a Modem

Unless you are lucky enough to be able to directly connect your computer to the Internet through an organization with which you are affiliated, your telecommunications activities will occur over telephone lines that connect your computer to other host computers. In addition to a telephone line, you will need a modem to translate messages passing back and forth between your computer and the line to which it is connected.

The primary feature of interest in a modem is its transmission speed, or baud rate. Generally speaking, you should purchase the fastest modem you can reasonably afford. As of this writing, the price and performance leader is a 14 400-baud modem, which can be purchased for as little as $75. The 28 800-baud modem is increasing in popularity and will soon be widely available. Remember, however, that no matter how fast your modem is, it will not transmit any faster than the capability of the modem on the other end. Therefore, if you are connecting to a service which uses only 9600 baud, then that is the maximum transmission speed. Despite this fact, if you can easily afford the faster modem, we recommend getting it. You will then be ready when your service upgrades.

If you have the opportunity, look for a recent review of different modems. Both PC and Macintosh magazines regularly review high-speed modems, and reading these updates can help you decide. Although transmission speed is the main factor, two modems of the same speed are not necessarily equal; sometimes one brand handles noisy lines better than the other, or one brand comes with a better warranty. You should also be aware that most modems come with generic communications programs which can be installed on your computer. If you choose to start out by connecting to bulletin board systems that do not provide you with customized software, then you can use the software included with your new modem to get started.

Getting on the Internet

This process can be a bit more challenging than connecting with the commercial vendors, but as the quality and quantity of useful medical information grow, it will become increasingly worth your effort.

If you are affiliated with a university or teaching hospital, or even some commercial organizations, Internet access may already be available to you. Staff in the computer department can give you more information on what kind of Internet access they can provide. Options can range from a direct connection to the Internet through the on-site network to a dial-up account that enables access from home and elsewhere.

Remember also, as we have noted earlier in this chapter, that nearly all of the value-added online service companies such as CompuServe, America Online, and Delphi offer some form of Internet access. Almost all offer access to e-mail messages, for example, but only a few offer access to the full range of Internet services. However, they too are getting caught up in "Internet fever," and many who do not currently offer full Internet functionality have plans to do so. Again, before you sign up with one of these vendors, ask them for a list of services they provide and are planning to provide in the near future.

If you would like to explore the Internet but do not have access through a university, commercial organization, or value-added service, try contacting an Internet provider in your area. Network providers, as they are known, allow persons to access the Internet by providing them with an "account." Some provide only limited access to services such as e-mail, but some enable access to a full range of Internet services. Additionally, some only allow access through a traditional dial-up connection, while a growing number allow access via the protocols known as SLIP or PPP (*see under* Connecting to Internet via Modem). Be sure to ask network providers for a list of Internet services you can access.

To find a local Internet provider (and to avoid long-distance charges when calling its network via modem), you should consult one of the Internet beginners' guides (for example, Prentice-Hall's *Internet: Getting Started*) for their extensive lists of local providers. You can also check the business pages of your local newspaper and the large, consumer-oriented computer magazines.

Connecting to Internet via Modem

The traditional method of connecting to the Internet involves logging onto a host computer already on the Internet and using your computer to exchange information with the host, which in turn carries out your instructions involving other Internet-connected computers. When you connect to the host via a high-speed network and use an appropriate communications protocol, you can rapidly exchange information across the entire Internet. Although you can use telephone lines and modems to connect to host computers on the Internet (at slower speeds than via a high-speed network), your computer and the host computer must communicate using an appropriate Internet protocol before you can use the rich Internet functionality. Two such communications protocols that allow your computer to connect to the Internet via modem are known as SLIP (Serial Line Internet Protocol) and PPP (Point to Point Protocol).

Some commercial and institutional providers of Internet connectivity are beginning to offer SLIP and PPP access. To use one of these protocols, appropriate software must be loaded both on your computer and on the host computer. While these protocols enable you to take advantage of Internet functionality beyond e-mail, transmission speeds are noticeably slower than with direct connections. This reduced performance can be especially noticeable when transferring large files such as multimedia material.

Starting to Use Internet Resources

A Master Resource

The Medical List is a database of Internet resources relevant to clinical medicine, which categorizes resources by disease, specialty, and other interest areas. Updated regularly, this database provides text descriptions of resources, spotlights the more developed programs, and gives news and background on Internet medical resource development. Currently, the file containing The Medical List prints out as roughly 85 pages. To obtain current information on accessing this resource, send an e-mail message to Dr. Gary Malet at "gmalet@surfer.win.net".

Discussion and Mailing Lists

An Internet mailing or discussion list is an easy way to get started on the Internet because all you need is the ability to send and receive e-mail from the Internet, not full connectivity. You simply send a message to a list that covers a topic of your interest (for example, clinical alerts), and the list automatically sends all the messages that it receives about that topic to your electronic mailbox. Remember that, if you use a commercial service that charges a fee to read each message from the Internet, these charges can quickly add up, especially on lists that send hundreds of messages a week. The following includes some Internet mailing lists that deal with computers in medicine.

FAM-MED. This mailing list discusses the use of computers in family medicine. To subscribe, send an e-mail message to "listproc@gac.edu". In the body of the message, type "subscribe fam-med" followed by your name. Leave the subject line blank.

HMATRIX-L. A discussion list about online health resources, it provides information about both Internet resources and electronic bulletin boards. To subscribe, send an e-mail message to "listserv@ ukanaix.cc.ukans.edu". In the body of the message, type "subscribe hmatrix-L" followed by your name. Leave the subject line blank.

HSPNET. This list was established for subscribers to discuss how hospitals can share data electronically, but much of the conversation is about the general use of computers and medicine. To subscribe, send an e-mail message to "listserv@albanydh2.bitnet". In the body of the message, type "subscribe hspnet-L" followed by your name. Leave the subject line blank. (Note that when using e-mail or URL addresses supplied in this book, the quotes should be omitted, and URLs are case-sensitive and should be entered exactly as they appear.)

Browsing through Medical Resources

If you have access to a browsing program such as Mosaic or Netscape (*see under* Mosaic: Multimedia and More), the following sites will show you some of the ways that medical information is being shared via the Internet. Each resource's address is called its URL, or universal resource locator, and directs the browsing program to the specified resource. Since browsing functionality provided by Mosaic and similar programs is relatively new, many of the available resources are considered to be "under construction," and thus their contents, links to other resources, and sometimes even their URLs can change unexpectedly.

HYPERDOC. This is the NLM's gateway to Internet medical resources, published by NLM and others (Figure 8-3). You can access it by using the following address: http://www.nlm.nih.gov/

ONCOLINK. This is the University of Pennsylvania's Multimedia Oncology Resource. You can access it by using the following address: http://cancer.med.upenn.edu/

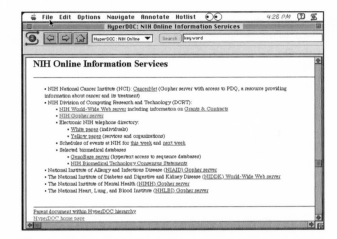

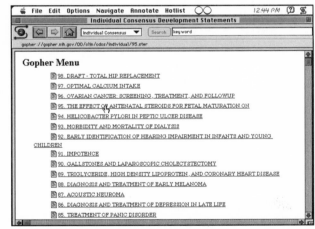

Figure 8-3. Screens within NLM's HyperDoc viewed through Mosaic. Top. A HyperDoc screen showing documents and servers that the user can access by selecting underlined items. **Bottom.** Partial menu of NIH Consensus Development Statements displayed when "NIH Gopher server" from the previous screen is selected. Full text of the statement is displayed when an underlined item from this screen is selected.

THE VIRTUAL HOSPITAL. This is a project of the University of Iowa College of Medicine, Department of Radiology. You can access it by using the following address: http://indy.radiology.uiowa.edu/Virtual Hospital.html

BREAST CANCER INFORMATION. This is maintained by the New York State Research and Education Network. You can access it by using the following address: http://nysernet.org/breast/Default.html

ONLINE MENDELIAN INHERITANCE IN MAN (OMIM). This is the online version of Victor McKusick's text. You can access it by using the following address: http://gdbwww.gdb.org/

Arriving with Telecommunications

Learning to telecommunicate brings a growing world of resources to your fingertips. For the rural physician, this technology can be a lifeline to stimulating dialogue in an area of special interest. For the academic physician, it provides a convenient way to collaborate with peers by sharing data regardless of geographic distance. No matter what category of physician you belong to, online capabilities can put you in touch with a growing body of current information available to assist you in managing your patients and in your continuing professional development. The potential uses of telecommunications discussed in this chapter will grow in scope as this technology matures. As transmission speeds increase and more people and institutions throughout our society become "connected," we will find ourselves using this method of communication and information access more and more in our daily lives.

9

CD-ROM Technology and Full-Text Information Retrieval

Jerome H. Carter, MD, FACP

HOW CAN CD-ROM TECHNOLOGY HELP ME IN MY PRACTICE?

For physicians, CD-ROM (compact disc–read-only memory) technology provides a wonderful solution to an old problem—staying current. Since the introduction of CD-ROM in 1982, advances in computer and information technologies have served to make it more affordable and easier to use. Estimates have been made that, as of 1994, over 11 million CD-ROM drives are in use in the United States, and over 6000 titles covering a wide range of topics are available on CD-ROM. The rise of CD-ROM as a reference and entertainment medium can readily be understood when one considers the storage capacity that each disc provides—680 Mb (680 million bytes). If that number is difficult to conceptualize, consider this: One 3.5-inch CD-ROM disc can hold the equivalent of 300 000 single-spaced, typewritten pages. Finally, any physician can own and easily access information that just a few years ago would have required a trip to the library.

Since having extensive information resources on hand for quick reference is a new experience for most practitioners, the effective and efficient use of these resources requires that the physician rethink his or her practice habits and information-seeking skills. The process of objectively and consistently monitoring your information needs and information-seeking behaviors is an important component of quality patient care because it serves to maintain the currency, depth, and breadth of your personal knowledge base.

CD-ROM technology, by making current information resources available at the point-of-care and by significantly reducing the time-costs involved in obtaining answers, has the ability to greatly reduce the problems many physicians have with managing their knowledge bases. CD-ROM technology is not a total solution, but it represents a significant advance in medical information management. It is affordable, approachable, and well worth the cost.

Improved Decision Making

The quality of any clinical decision is based on two factors: the physician's judgment and the information available about the problem at hand. The breadth of information that goes into even the simplest patient encounter is quite amazing. Caring for a patient with dysuria requires familiarity with diseases (cystitis, pyelonephritis, renal stones) and drugs (indications, spectrum, side effects, interactions). For example, a 35-year-old woman who recently moved to the United States from Sicily presents with a complaint of dysuria for the last 3 days. Which drug regimen would be most appropriate for this patient? What particular sensitivities might she have? Until the advent of CD-ROM, getting all the pertinent information would have required a good deal of page turning. Now, various new products make it possible to consult several reference sources in a few seconds, resulting in more authoritative decisions made with greater confidence.

WHAT CD-ROM PRODUCTS ARE AVAILABLE NOW?

CD-ROM medical reference titles are available in three primary forms: books, full-text journals, and journal citations. Increasingly, CD-ROM–based continuing medical education (CME) programs (either stand-alone programs or bundled with CD-ROM–based references) are becoming available (*see* Chapter 7). In addition, other types of multi-application CD-ROMs are being released. For example, First DataBank offers a single disk that has a diagnostic support program (QMR; *see* Chapter 4), a drug information program (Ask Rx; *see* Chapter 5), and a patient education program (Ask Advice; *see* Chapter 6). Other examples of multipurpose discs are described later in this chapter.

To better understand the discussion of the specific programs available on CD-ROM, you need to have some knowledge of the relation between the CD-ROM drive and the computer system. Buying CD-ROM drives and titles requires some familiarity with computer-industry jargon and a few technical concepts. A basic knowledge of these topics will save you time and money and prevent the frustration usually associated with buying computer products.

Hardware Interfaces

The interface is the communication path between the CD-ROM drive and the computer. Three types of interfaces are available: proprietary, small computer systems interfaces (SCSI), and parallel.

PROPRIETARY INTERFACES. These are sold with the CD-ROM drive and are made only by the drive manufacturer. They tend to be fast and will definitely work with the CD-ROM drive. In addition, they are relatively inexpensive. On the down side, they will not work with a CD-ROM drive from a different manufacturer, and they may also be difficult to install. Unless you like to do-it-yourself and upgrade equipment often, you should avoid proprietary interfaces.

SMALL COMPUTER SYSTEMS INTERFACES (SCSI). These are industry-standard interfaces that work with various computer components. SCSI (pronounced "scuzzy") interfaces for CD-ROM drives are available from several manufacturers. They are usually easier to install than proprietary interfaces and work with CD-ROM drives from different companies. They are the most flexible of the three interface types and are highly recommended.

PARALLEL INTERFACES. These connect to your computer through the same port as does the printer. They are the slowest type of interface but by far the easiest to set up. They may be the only viable choice for use with some portable computers.

Drives

The selection of CD-ROM drives has markedly improved in recent months. Costs have steadily declined while performance has quadrupled. Four categories of drives are currently available: portable, external, internal, and disc changers.

PORTABLE DRIVES. For those who come to depend on CD-ROM references, portable drives are a marvelous invention. They are distinguished from other drive types by the fact that they may be operated using batteries and are easily carried in a briefcase or portable computer case. In terms of performance, they rank slightly below other drives.

EXTERNAL DRIVES. These are the forebears of portable drives. They offer little advantage over the best portable drives because they are heavier, less flexible, and require AC power. They are, however, slightly faster than portables.

INTERNAL DRIVES. These are installed inside the computer much as are floppy-disk drives. They are the least expensive type of drive. However, since they are housed inside the computer unit, flexibility is low (if you buy another computer, you cannot move the drive to the new system as easily as you could a portable or external drive). Internal drives are becoming the most common type because many computer manufacturers are installing them at the factory. If saving money is your chief objective when buying a drive, internal is the way to go.

DISC CHANGERS. Capacity is the main selling point for disc changers. These "juke box" drives can hold six or more CD-ROM discs at once. While this can be a convenient arrangement, frequent switching between discs can be time consuming, and these drives allow access to only one CD at a time.

Multisession Discs and Photo CDs

Until recently, CD-ROM discs were always created at one "printing" session. Thus, if you were going to put a textbook on disc, the entire book would have to be placed on the disc in one session. If you wished to add another chapter a year later, an entirely new disc would have to be created—material could not be added to the original disc once it was printed (or pressed). These discs may be referred to as single-session discs. Recently, manufacturers found a way to add information to a disc long after it had been printed. Such discs are called multisession discs.

Photo CD refers to a technology pioneered by Kodak and Philips Corporation. These discs are used to store digitized photographic images (35 mm). Photo CDs can have images added to them at different times, which makes them a specialized kind of multisession disc.

All CD-ROM drives are not capable of reading multi-session discs. Be sure to check for this feature on drives, if you think you may want the ability to read photo CDs or other multisession discs.

Retrieval Software

Specially designed software is needed to access the information on a CD-ROM disc. The retrieval software comes bundled with the CD and is specific for that product. Thus, if you make use of multiple CD reference sources, you will probably have to learn how to use multiple programs. Retrieval software is composed of two basic components: the search engine and the user interface.

Search Engine

The ability to do fast, detailed searches through a large amount of text is the main feature that has led to the rapid acceptance of CD-ROM as a reference medium. The search engine is the part of the software that retrieves different passages from the reference text, depending on your input. Search engines usually provide for several different kinds of searches, each suited to a specific type of information need.

TABLE OF CONTENTS SEARCHES. Perhaps the simplest type of search is via the table of contents (also referred to as browsing). Searching in this manner is similar to using a book's table of contents. From a list of available topics, you select one for viewing.

TEXT-WORD SEARCHES. Text-word searches are more complex and illustrate well the wonders of CD-ROM. A typical text-word search for the word "hypothyroidism" would result in the retrieval of all occurrences of the text word from the entire database, regardless of the relevance of the findings. If this search were done using an internal medicine textbook, many references of marginal value would be returned. Search engines, however, provide the ability to do Boolean searches using logical operators such as AND, OR, and NOT (for example, hypothyroidism AND effusion) to expand or restrict the possible findings according to the searcher's preference.

PHRASE-BASED SEARCHES. Some products allow the fine-tuning of text-word searches by using phrase-based searches and proximity rules. Phrase searches are useful when only exact matches are desired. "Hypothyroidism after radioactive iodine therapy" is an example of a phrase-based search. Using this type of search inappropriately is often frustrating because few matches are likely. This type of search should never be used as an initial search strategy.

PROXIMITY SEARCHES. Proximity searches provide an additional means of adjusting the specificity of a search. They are more forgiving than phrase-based searches and may be used as an initial query type. In general, search engines that support proximity searches allow you to specify the maximum distance between two keywords in the item being searched.

User Interfaces

The user interface is the program component you interact with; it accepts your input and displays the results of your search. The interface may be graphical (Macintosh or Windows) or character based (DOS or UNIX). Ease of use is a major issue in determining if a particular interface is suitable for you. Note that ease of use is not limited to a particular type of interface (that is, graphical interfaces may be difficult to learn and character-based ones may be easy). Most products mentioned in this chapter have well-designed interfaces, so ease of use may not be a major concern. Besides ease-of-use factors, other functions—for example, stored search histories—provided by the interface may make a particular product better in terms of its productivity and flexibility.

STORED SEARCH HISTORIES. Of the more common functions found in interface software, stored search histories are without a doubt the most useful. Each time you perform a search, the software keeps track of the search terms and results; this is referred to as a search history. If you wish to repeat the search in the future, you need only activate the old search. The true value of this feature is seen in products that are frequently updated because it directly addresses the problem of staying current. Using stored search histories, it is easier for you to keep up with the latest in your field. You simply run the stored search against the update disc, and all new information pertaining to that query is automatically retrieved.

Books Available on CD-ROM

PDR (Physician's Desk Reference) on CD-ROM

PDR on CD-ROM is a drug-information reference containing text from the following sources: *Physician's Desk Reference; PDR for Ophthalmology; PDR for Nonprescription Drugs;* and *PDR Guide to Drug Interactions, Side Effects and Indications.* The retrieval software for PDR on CD-ROM supports all basic and advanced search features as well as text exporting and stored histories. Other than the standard information one expects from the *PDR,* many special features are offered that enhance the value of the product. For example, the program allows look-up of drugs by indication, side effect, therapeutic category, and drug interaction. The drug-interaction function accepts multi-drug regimens and stores patient information for future use. Annual updates are provided. The *Merck Manual* is available as an option with PDR on CD-ROM and uses the PDR retrieval software.

MAXX: Maximum Access to Diagnosis and Therapy

MAXX consists of 24 titles from the Spiral Manual series published by Little, Brown and Company. Titles from pediatrics, gynecology, neurology, dermatology, emergency medicine, and all subspecialties of internal medicine are offered. Additionally, drug and laboratory information references are provided. Some examples of the titles available on MAXX are Manual of Medical Therapeutics, A Pocket Manual of

Differential Diagnosis, Manual of Cardiovascular Diagnosis and Therapy, Manual of Endocrinology and Metabolism, and A Practical Approach to Infectious Diseases. MAXX's retrieval software supports all basic and advanced search features with the

Figure 9-1. STAT!-Ref. Top. Search screen shows five searchable book titles that have been licensed by a user from the STAT!-Ref primary care library. Note that the user is searching for BPH (benign prostatic hypertrophy) and PSA (prostate specific antigen) in all these texts. **Bottom.** Beginning of results screen showing the outcome of the search.

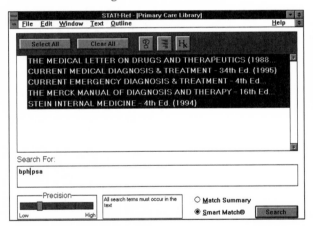

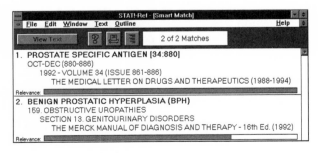

exception of proximity searches. Stored searches are supported, but text exporting is not. Quarterly updates are provided.

STAT!-Ref

STAT!-Ref is perhaps the most ambitious of all CD-ROM titles currently available. It provides a library of 27 textbooks covering topics in internal medicine, surgery, pediatrics, obstetrics and gynecology, emergency medicine, drug information, and practice guidelines. Ten years of MEDLINE citations from 20 journals are also included in the basic package. Figure 9-1 shows a search and a results screen. Focused subscriptions are offered in primary care, cardiology, and oncology, with each containing a different combination of textbooks and journals. STAT!-Ref offers more sophisticated retrieval software compared with several other CD-ROM medical reference titles, which means more capability and, for some, a steeper learning curve. All basic and advanced search features are supported. The manual is quite good and must be read if one is to master the software. Quarterly updates are provided.

Scientific American Medicine on CD-ROM (SAM-CD)

SAM-CD is an electronic version of the popular monthly updated textbook *Scientific American Medicine* and covers all areas of internal medicine as well as dermatology, neurology, and psychiatry (Figure 9-2). As a bonus, CME credits are offered via the DISCOTEST series. SAM-CD retrieval software supports text export and all basic and advanced search features except stored searches. Its full-color graphics greatly enhance the value of the product. SAM-CD has the fastest search engine of all the textbooks reviewed. Quarterly updates are provided.

Clinical Dermatology Illustrated: A Regional Approach

Clinical Dermatology is one of a number of medical reference products published by Continuing Medical Education Associates. Aimed at primary care physicians, this product provides diagnostic algorithms, treatment information, and full-color photographs for common skin lesions. Also included are audio snippets from lectures by the book's authors. Only basic search functions are provided. No export or stored search capabilities are supported.

PrimePractice

PrimePractice is an ambitious product produced by the Mayo Clinic with IVI Publishing. It represents the next step in the evolution of CD-ROM–based medical references, making excellent use of full-motion video, sound, and superb color graphics. PrimePractice is based on the Mayo Clinic's board review materials and is produced quarterly as a series of CDs dedicated to a particular subspecialty topic. The initial offering covers cardiology topics. The case studies provided allow interactive patient encounters during which one can listen to heart sounds and respirations, rotate the patient, and so forth. However, all of these wonderful multimedia features come at a price. In order to use these CDs effectively, you need a 486 computer (33 MHz or higher), at least 8 Mb of

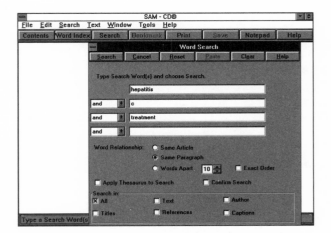

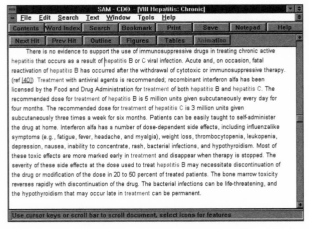

Figure 9-2. SAM-CD. Top. Search screen with search for "hepatitis c treatment." **Bottom.** Some of the text found by the search. Note the highlighted search terms in the text.

RAM, a sound card, speakers, and a double-speed CD drive. The search engine provided allows Boolean but not proximity searches. Also, text exporting is limited. Bookmarks are supported. Unfortunately, the update policy is not in keeping with those of other CD title providers. As of this writing, PrimePractice titles will not be updated until a complete cycle of all subspecialty titles has been published. In other words, the cardiology CD may not be updated for 2 years or more.

Journal Citations Available on CD-ROM

STAT!-Ref

As mentioned earlier, STAT!-Ref provides MEDLINE citations and abstracts for up to the past 10 years from selected journals. The material is grouped by discipline. At present, offerings are available for primary care, oncology, and cardiology.

Aries Knowledge Finder

Aries Systems Corporation provides a comprehensive set of literature databases covering all areas of medicine. Of particular note is Aries Knowledge Finder, a unique implementation of retrieval software which allows natural language searches (for example, "Is hypothyroidism associated with congestive heart failure?"). The basic product offered is an unabridged version of MEDLINE (1966 to present) covering 3500 journals and is updated quarterly. Specialty-oriented versions of Knowledge Finder are offered in cardiology, primary care, neurology, obstetrics and gynecology, ophthalmology, orthopedics, pathology, pediatrics, radiology, surgery, and AIDS. Stored searches are supported; text exporting is not.

SilverPlatter Information, Inc.

SilverPlatter products cover a wide range of topics in many professional fields. Databases from the National Library of Medicine are offered (that is, MEDLINE, AIDSLINE, CancerLit, TOXLINE) as well as the complete set of Excerpta Medica, which provides topic-specific bibliographic databases in areas such as cardiology, obstetrics and gynecology, pathology, neurosciences, psychiatry, anesthesiology, and so on, with each database covering 10 or more years of citations. SilverPlatter's retrieval software, called SPIRS, provides numerous basic and advanced functions.

Full-Text Journals Available on CD-ROM

Appleton & Lange New Media

Appleton & Lange New Media (formerly Macmillan New Media) offers The New England Journal of Medicine, Annals of Internal Medicine, Journal of the American Medical Association, The Lancet, and British Medical Journal in full-text versions. They are provided in two ways: as a 1-year grouping of all five journals or as a multi-year CD of just one journal. The retrieval software supports basic and advanced search features and stored search histories. No text exporting is permitted. In addition to its full-text offerings, Appleton & Lange also offers MEDLINE citation databases and AIDS articles and textbooks on CD.

Creative Multimedia Corporation Research

Creative Multimedia offers full-text renditions of The New England Journal of Medicine, American Family Physician, Pediatrics, Pediatric Infectious Disease Journal, and selected titles from the Mosby-Yearbook, Inc., series. Only basic search functions are provided. No export or stored search capabilities are supported.

Table 9-1 lists the CD-ROM products and vendors discussed in this chapter. Further information on these and other products can be found in various catalogs and product reviews (see Appendix).

HOW CAN I IMPLEMENT CD-ROM TECHNOLOGY IN MY PRACTICE?

The most important factors to take into account when you are trying to decide if CD-ROM technology is right for you are your information needs (current and future) and your practice characteristics. Once you have decided that your information and practice needs would be met by CD-ROM technology, the next steps are simple. You should review or look into some of the basic issues pertaining to purchase, set-up, and hardware. The technology is easy to understand and is available from a number of vendors.

Information Needs

If you see patients on a regular basis, you need access to timely information. Medical references on CD-ROM are excellent tools for addressing information needs that arise during patient care because a vast collection of resources can be easily searched and updated. Do not fall into the trap of thinking that "I do not use reference sources very often now, so my information needs are being met." Why? Many physicians are not adept at recognizing when they have unmet needs. Having better access to useful information sources may improve the recognition and resolution of these needs.

Practice Characteristics

PRACTICE HABITS. If you find that you frequently obtain consults for reasons other than procedures or difficult cases, lack of timely information might be the cause. Also, if detailed documentation of diagnostic and therapeutic strategies is desired, or if providing your patients with the latest information on their health problems is important to you, CD-ROM will appeal to you. Finally, if searching for medical information at home is practical and you are considering purchasing (or already own) a home computer, you might consider using medical CD-ROMs there. The rapid growth in home usage of education and

Table 9-1. CD-ROM Medical Reference Products Discussed

Products	Type of Publication	Platform	Price*	Publisher or Manufacturer	Address	Phone and Fax Numbers
American Family Physician, Pediatrics, others	Full-text journals, books	Macintosh, Windows	$$-$$$	Creative Multimedia Corporation Research	322 N.W. Fifth Avenue Suite 201 Portland, OR 97209	Tel: 800-854-9126 503-242-2567 Fax: 503-242-0519
Clinical Dermatology Illustrated	Book	DOS, Macintosh, Windows	$$	Continuing Medical Education Associates	P.O. Box 109074 Chicago, IL 60610	Tel: 800-227-CMEA Fax: 312-733-3107
Aries Knowledge Finder	Journal citations	DOS, Macintosh, Windows	$$-$$$$	Aries Systems Corporation	200 Sutton Street North Andover, MA 01845	Tel: 508-975-7570 Fax: 508-975-3811
NEJM, Annals, JAMA, Lancet, BMJ, Textbook of AIDS Medicine	Full-text journals, books	DOS, Macintosh, Windows	$$-$$$	Appleton & Lange New Media	P.O. Box 5630 Norwalk, CT 06856	Tel: 800-423-1359 Fax: 203-854-9486
MAXX: Maximum Access to Diagnosis and Therapy	Books	Macintosh, Windows	$$-$$$$	Little, Brown and Company	34 Beacon Street Boston, MA 02108	Tel: 800-289-6299 617-859-5549 Fax: 617-859-0629
Physicians' SilverPlatter MEDLINE	Journal citations	DOS, Macintosh, Windows	$$-$$$	SilverPlatter Information, Inc.	100 River Ridge Drive Norwood, MA 02062	Tel: 800-289-6299 617-769-2599 Fax: 617-769-8763
PDR on CD-ROM	Book	DOS	$$$	Medical Economics Data	5 Paragon Drive Montvale, NJ 07645	Tel: 800-232-7379 Fax: 201-573-4956
PrimePractice	Books	Macintosh, Windows	$$	IVI Publishing	7500 Flying Cloud Drive Minneapolis, MN 55435	Tel: 800-661-6170
SAM-CD	Book	DOS, Macintosh, Windows	$$-$$$	Scientific American Medicine	415 Madison Avenue New York, NY 10017	Tel: 800-545-0544 212-754-0801 Fax: 212-980-3062
STAT!-Ref	Books, journal citations	Macintosh, Windows	$$-$$$$	Teton Data Systems	P.O. Box 3082 Jackson, WY 83001	Tel: 800-755-7828 307-733-5494 Fax: 307-739-1229

* $=under $100; $$=$101 to $500; $$$=$501 to $1000; $$$$=over $1000. Prices are approximate at the time of printing.

entertainment CD-ROMs may make this a relatively painless way to get started.

PRACTICE LOCATION. If you are office-based or in a rural area, CD-ROM provides you with access to a wealth of resources with minimal inconvenience. Even physicians who spend most of their time in a hospital setting may find the point-of-care convenience afforded by CD-ROM appealing. Relatively few such institutions provide access to medical resources on CD-ROM, but the number is growing.

PRACTICE SIZE. The cost of implementing CD-ROM, while not oppressive, is not insignificant. Therefore, the larger the practice, the easier it is to absorb the cost—presuming, of course, that you and your partners can agree on what kind of computer and which software titles to buy.

CURRENT LEVEL OF AUTOMATION. Practices that currently use computers for non-business purposes will find it easier to implement CD-ROM technology from the standpoint of price and possibly location. If computers in your practice are already fully utilized for billing and other management functions and it is not possible to easily redirect their usage, new systems will be needed. Also, most dedicated business machines are not located in areas of the office that would make them useful for point-of-care information retrieval. Computers used for clinical purposes are usually in good locations and are probably underutilized by the medical staff; therefore, they are excellent candidates for use with CD-ROMs.

PRACTICE TYPE. Most CD-ROM offerings (especially full-text references) are aimed at generalist and primary-care physicians. Thus, for the foreseeable future, the greatest benefit can be expected to accrue to internists, family practitioners, and emergency-medicine specialists. However, excellent coverage of subspecialty topics is available via bibliographic citation products.

Purchase and Set-up Issues

Once you have decided that you want to invest in CD-ROM technology, turning your attention to technical and business matters becomes necessary.

COMPUTER TYPE. This part is simple. If you already have computers in your practice, then use one of them or purchase another of the same type. The only exception I would offer concerns multimedia. Multimedia refers to CD-ROMs that provide full-motion video, sound, or animation, or all three, in one CD. Currently, Macintosh computers offer a lot more than IBM-compatibles in the way of built-in features supporting multimedia applications. And should you ever decide to experiment, the Macintosh is a much friendlier computer for do-it-yourself projects.

OTHER HARDWARE. Monitors, printers, and other computer peripherals are well supported by all computer types currently on the market. You may shop based purely on value for these items.

CD-ROM DRIVES. In general, get the fastest drive you can afford and, if at all possible, a SCSI interface. Further discussion of CD-ROM drives is given in Hardware Issues later in this chapter.

CD-ROM CONFIGURATION. Your CD-ROM drive may be set up as a stand-alone unit connected to a single computer or connected to several computers on a network. If you are in a large practice (for example, a group or clinic), networked drives may be more cost-effective for providing access to all practitioners. Remember, however, that the price for using CD-ROM software increases when used on a network.

Software Issues

A disconcerting discovery for many first-time CD users is that CD-ROM software is sold as a subscription much like a magazine. Therefore, every year you must repay all or a percentage of the original purchase price to maintain the currency of the software. This fact must be accounted for when budgeting for CD-ROM products. Some vendors actually program their CD-ROM software to disable itself after expiration of the license if you do not renew your subscription. Fortunately, this practice is disappearing.

CD-ROMs are superior to print reference sources for two reasons: They provide fast access to large amounts of information, and most are updated on a quarterly basis. Thus, they are out-of-date much less often than standard print references. These advantages do not come without a price. More than likely, your annual expenditure on information resources will increase from previous expenditures on print-based sources.

Hardware Issues

No prior experience is necessary to make full use of CD-ROM. Installation of all required peripherals can be arranged by your vendor, and the manuals from your CD-ROM player and your computer oper-ating system should be enough to get you started. If you are completely computer illiterate or computer phobic, you should carefully consider buying a Macintosh, since they are closest to "plug and play."

Hardware Layout

Your first major decision will be hardware layout. In other words, will you be using your CD with a portable or desktop computer, at home or at your office? If you are in solo practice, a portable computer provides the most flexible setup. In a large group, a network setup is more cost-effective.

Where will your computer be used? This point is minor but could save you a lot of money. Computers suitable for use at home cost much less and often have CD-ROM drives preinstalled at a significant cost advantage over business systems. Also, they perform well enough that you are unlikely to notice any problems. A system designed for use at home is also good for office use, provided that it will never be needed for use on a network or other serious business functions. An additional consideration is your information-seeking behavior. There seem to be at least two information-seeking patterns: "immediate look up" and "save for later." If you fall into the latter group, then a home-based system might be your best bet. The explosion of CD-ROM titles (games, encyclopedias, and so on), many of which are bundled with drives, make home usage an even more attractive option for many clinicians.

Buying Hardware

SELECTING A VENDOR. The most important concerns when selecting a retail vendor are location, service, cost, and, of course, quality. Many large chains (for example, CompUSA and Micro Center) sell "house-brand" IBM-compatibles that are very reliable, inexpensive, and of high quality. These chains usually provide quality service and warranty packages as well as good, basic computer training courses. A selection of mail-order catalogs offer a variety of software and hardware at a discount (*see* Appendix, Chapter 11). When selecting a CD-ROM drive, I suggest staying with the major manufacturers. CD-ROM hardware is frequently reviewed in popular computer magazines, which are a valuable source of up-to-date comparative information. Personally, I am fond of NEC drives for several reasons, including their good warranty, support of all industry standards, and easy-to-use interface.

COMPUTER TYPE. Buy a computer similar to the type you already own; this lessens support problems and learning time. If you do not currently own a computer, then shop with an eye toward price and features.

BUYING A CD-ROM DRIVE. Before you set out to buy a drive, you should understand the following terms: access time and transfer rate. The access time refers to the time it takes the drive to locate requested information on the disc. Most drives have access times between 250 and 800 milliseconds. The lower the number, the better. Never buy a drive with an access time of greater than 500 milliseconds. The transfer rate is a measurement of how quickly the drive can move information from the disc to your computer's memory. The base transfer rate for drives currently available is 150 Kb/sec. Recently, advances in CD-ROM technology have resulted in drives with much faster transfer rates. The availability of drives with faster transfer rates has changed the way this feature is referred to within the computer industry. Drives that transfer information at the 150 Kb/sec rate are now referred to as single-speed drives; those that operate at 300 Kb/sec are called double-speed drives, and at 450 Kb/sec, they are called triple-speed drives. Most recently, quadruple-speed drives have become available. For reference use, double-speed drives are more than adequate. If you are thinking about using multimedia applications, however, faster is better.

DRIVE TYPE. Internal drives tend to be less expensive than portable or external drives, and portable drives are the most flexible. External drives have no good selling points. If price is an issue, get an internal drive; if not, get a portable one. Either type may be used on a network. (*See under* Drives earlier in this chapter for further discussion of drive types.)

BUS INTERFACE. A SCSI is the best choice for an interface. If price is an issue, you may save a little by buying a proprietary interface. (*See under* Hardware Interfaces earlier in this chapter for further discussion.)

NETWORKS. Most network operating systems work well with CD-ROM drives. Therefore, this should not be a concern.

INSTALLATION AND SUPPORT. Portable drives that use parallel interfaces are easily installed by anyone with minimal computer experience. If you must install a card inside the computer (for example, if you buy a drive for a desktop computer that uses a SCSI or proprietary interface), then have your vendor do it. You have better things to do with your time. Note that because Macintosh computers use built-in SCSI interfaces for peripherals, installation is usually very easy for these systems. Support for your drive comes from the manufacturer, so choose well. Drives from Chinon, NEC, and Apple have received excellent reviews in computer-industry magazines, although excellent drives are available from a number of manufacturers.

Buying CD-ROM Titles

Caveat emptor: Many (but not all) titles are available for both Macintosh and IBM-compatible computers. If you do not already have a computer but are planning to buy one, the availability of CD-ROM titles you are likely to want may affect your decision. Of course, when buying a CD-ROM title, you must make sure you are getting a version that runs on your platform. Similarly, you must make sure your computer is appropriately equipped for sound and video processing if you are interested in using multimedia titles.

The general recommendations for selecting hardware and software discussed in the Introduction to this book may be especially helpful in selecting CD-ROM titles that will be most useful to you. Installation for all packages mentioned in this chapter is straightforward, so this should not be a concern. The major point to remember when selecting a CD-ROM title is that you are purchasing a subscription, and therefore, you will be required to pay an annual fee that is equal to, or a significant percentage of, the original purchase price.

Overall, the hardware and software are affordable, and the advances made possible by CD-ROM technology allow you to make great strides in your ability to access and manage medical information. Once you become comfortable accessing medical information on CD-ROM, you will probably wonder how you coped without this technology.

10

PORTABLE COMPUTING DEVICES

Donald L. Vine, MD, FACP

. . . .

HOW CAN PORTABLE COMPUTING DEVICES HELP ME IN MY PRACTICE?

Physicians are expected to retain and accurately process an unbelievable amount of information. While portable computing will not eliminate these expectations, available technology can make them easier to meet. Clinicians, frequently on the run, gather many scraps of information and face the challenge of effectively saving, organizing, and retrieving them. Portable computing offers numerous advantages over conventional methods of managing the daily onslaught of miscellaneous data. Four points of special interest to the medical practitioner are discussed in the following section.

Advantages of Portable Computing

Flexible Entering and Organizing of New Information

The most obvious use of portable computing is for managing scraps of information such as appointments, telephone numbers, meeting reminders, anniversary events, and so forth. These short pieces of text are often associated with a date and time. Somewhat lengthier material (for example, travel instructions, agendas, and even presentation outlines) can also be readily managed.

Any piece of information with an associated telephone number may represent an important or useful contact and be potentially valuable. Did you ever hear at a hospital staff meeting that a new third-party reviewer was changing some rules? If you had written down the name and number of the person presenting the information, plus a few key words, you could quickly locate help to recall this information months after you had forgotten the name of the source. Or perhaps you did jot it down on a scratch pad and now have no idea what happened to that piece of paper.

Expenses, odometer readings, time spent with patients, and billing codes are examples of notes with associated quantities that can be used for personal tax records or by your office staff for preparation of patient charges and third-party documentation. Here again, the portable computer permits you to enter the information on the run and use it whenever and wherever you need it.

The intelligent use of portable computers also reduces the chore of organizing miscellaneous information recorded throughout the day. If you were to record the name and telephone number of every person you called and the company name and number from every advertisement or product announcement that interested you, then the time spent capturing such information would be offset by the increased organization, retrievability, and security of these details. And the more compulsively you enter such random notes, the more useful your portable computer becomes.

Immediate Availability of Reference Information

Currently, you can carry up to 80 Mb (80 million characters), or about 46 000 typed pages, of information in electronic format in your pocket. A wealth of medical material is available for use on portable devices. Each month, you can download abstracts from your favorite three or four journals and review them between patient visits, using your pocket computer as a book. Alternatively, you can transfer selections from *Scientific American Medicine* or one of the many *Yearbooks* and review the material whenever and wherever you have a few moments.

Add to this a drug interaction program, key information about each of your patients, selected guidelines, and other key clinical references—and you may still have room for more (for example, the names, addresses, and telephone numbers of everyone currently listed in your personal address book).

Information that is not immediately available within the memory of the hand-held device can be obtained using a portable modem and a telephone from commercial databases such as CompuServe, CDP Colleague, and the National Library of Medicine. Hospital and office databases can be configured to permit the same kind of data exchange. Using available wireless technology, you can affordably capture health news and stock quotes as well as messages from your office.

Faster and More Complete Data Entry than by Hand

There is a body of literature that says the use of symptom-related forms and checklists provides superior patient care because details are not omitted. Forms and checklists directly related to patient symptoms lend themselves well to portable computing; they can be carried in your pocket or on a small, portable device.

While hand-held devices are not yet suitable for translating speech into a history of the present illness, the symptom-directed review of systems, past medical history, and much of the physical examination can be completed using a checklist in your computer. A good set of checklists reduces the time required to collect information to document your patients' progress and responses to treatment. If a summary of each hospitalization or visit is perceived as a piece of tomorrow's past medical history, these "random" pieces of patient information quickly become a useful part of each patient's medical record.

Prompt Communication of Data to Others

Combine a portable computer with a fax/modem, and you can send correspondence, clinical data, or other information almost anywhere, almost instantly, from wherever you are, as long as there is a telephone hookup. Using well-chosen hardware and software, you could send a final consultation report to a referring doctor's office shortly after you leave a patient or complete a procedure.

With some devices, you can save drawings to use for patient education. With others, you can present a slide show to students and residents.

WHAT TYPES OF PORTABLE COMPUTING PRODUCTS ARE AVAILABLE?

With advancing computer technology, an increasing variety of new-generation, small, battery-powered portable devices can be found. Like the technology itself, the terminology is in flux, and devices referred to by some as *pocket* computers are described by others as *palmtops*. The palmtops are often associated with pen-enabled computers, which may be marketed as PDAs, or *personal digital assis-*

tants. The term *laptop* was used a few years ago to describe any small, full-keyboard computer that could conveniently be placed on your lap; smaller versions of the same came to be called *notebook* computers because they could fit in your briefcase. Currently, ultra-lightweight *subnotebooks* are extremely popular.

For the purposes of selecting equipment, you can reasonably assume that a device that weighs more than 3 pounds or runs less than 4 hours on a single battery charge is not likely to be a constant portable companion. With that in mind, the major determinant of size for your purchase should be whether you need a full-sized keyboard, commercial PC software, or pen-based data entry; you can then divide portable personal computing devices into these three broad classes (mindful of the terminology blur affecting the whole market):

1. Palmtop, or pocket, devices that can be held comfortably in the hand, or, at the smaller end, that weigh less than 7 ounces and fit comfortably in a pocket or small purse

2. PDAs or pen-compatible computers, usually with a pen-sensitive drawing surface and a size too large to fit comfortably into a pocket

3. Subnotebooks, ultra-lightweight computers with "full-sized" keyboards and a hinged display lid.

This chapter discusses some selected product examples of portable computers from these three categories. Table 10-1 provides more information about those products. Since new products are introduced into this growing market every month, interested readers should pursue the subject by browsing through computer magazines or visiting an electronics or computer store. The features you should

Table 10-1. Portable Computing Products Discussed

Type of Computer, Product	Platform	Price*	Name and Address of Manufacturer	Phone and Fax Numbers
Palmtops				
Franklin Digital Book System	Proprietary system	$-$$	Franklin Electronic Publishers, Inc. 122 Burrs Road Mt. Holly, NJ 08060	Tel: 800-762-5382 609-261-4800 Fax: 609-261-1631
HP 200 LX Palmtop PC	DOS	$$$	Hewlett-Packard 1000 N.E. Circle Boulevard Corvallis, OR 97330	Tel: 800-443-1254 503-715-3141 Fax: 503-715-3008
Psion 3a	Proprietary system	$$-$$$	Psion 150 Baker Avenue Concord, MA 01742	Tel: 800-774-6697 Fax: 508-371-9611
Wizard Organizer	Proprietary system	$$	Sharp Electronics Box 8, Sharp Plaza Mahwah, NJ 07430	Tel: 800-237-4277 Fax: 201-512-2045
Personal digital assistants				
Newton Message Pad 110	Proprietary system	$$$	Apple Computers, Inc. 1 Infinite Loop Cupertino, CA 95014	Tel: 800-767-2775 Fax: 408-996-1010
Tandy Zoomer	Windows	$$	Radio Shack 1500 One Tandy Center Fort Worth, TX 76102	Tel: 817-390-3205 Fax: 817-390-3217

* $=under $100; $$=$101 to $500; $$$=$501 to $1000; $$$$=over $1000. Prices are approximate at the time of printing.
† For information on Apple Macintosh notebook computers, contact Apple Computers, Inc., at 800-767-2775.

evaluate when shopping for portable computers include the category of the device (as above), weight and size, screen size, type and life of the battery, processor speed, available RAM and hard-drive capacity, and price. You should also consider Personal Computer Memory Card International Association (PCMCIA) compatibility, as described in the following section.

Memory Cards

Before considering which type of portable computer to buy, you must understand how these devices handle memory and storage capacity. Many portable computers use a device roughly the size of a credit card that serves as the equivalent of a hard-disk drive. A widely used standard for these devices, also known as cards, is the PCMCIA standard. Most portable devices that accept cards can handle PCMCIA cards; notable exceptions include the Psion 3a and Franklin Digital Books (*see under* Pocket or Palmtop Computers), both of which use their own proprietary memory-card format.

PCMCIA cards are designated as either type I, type II, or type III. Depending on the card and the portable device, type I and II cards can be used as

Table 10-1. (*Continued*)

Type of Computer, Product	Platform	Price*	Name and Address of Manufacturer	Phone and Fax Numbers
Subnotebooks†				
Compaq Aero	DOS, Windows	$$$-$$$$	Compaq Computer Corp. Mail Code 110302 20555 State Hwy. 249 Houston, TX 77070	Tel: 800-888-5858 Fax: 800-888-5329 Contact: Brian Allen
Gateway 2000 Handbook	DOS, Windows	$$$-$$$$	Gateway P.O. Box 2000 610 Gateway Drive North Sioux City, SD 57049	Tel: 800-846-2000 Fax: 605-232-2023
HP Omni 530	DOS, Windows	$$$$	Hewlett-Packard 1000 N.E. Circle Boulevard Corvallis, OR 97330	Tel: 800-443-1254 503-715-3141 Fax: 503-715-3008
IBM ThinkPad 510	DOS, Windows	$$$$	IBM 2039 Cornwallis Road Research Triangle Park, NC 27709	Tel: 800-426-3333 Fax: 800-426-4182
Toshiba Portégé	DOS, Windows	$$$$	Toshiba 9740 Irvine Boulevard Irvine, CA 92713	Tel: 800-631-3811 Fax: 714-587-6648
Zenith Z-Lite 425L, Model 170W	DOS, Windows	$$$$	Zenith Data Systems 2150 E. Lake Cook Road Buffalo Grove, IL 60089	Tel: 800-533-0331 Fax: 800-472-7211

ROM (for example, when a reference text comes preloaded and unchangeable on the card), as RAM, or as a storage device (for example, similar to a hard-disk drive). PCMCIA ROM cards tend to be less expensive than cards that allow information to be stored as well as retrieved.

Some cards use a static charge to maintain information stored for up to 5 years without any battery backup. Other types of cards require a battery to maintain the stored information, but these tend to store and retrieve information faster. PCMCIA cards currently come in data capacities of up to 40 Mb. Data-compression software available for some devices—for example, Hewlett Packards, Newtons,

and subnotebooks—can double the usable capacity. As the storage capacity of the type II cards increases, the price approaches, and may even exceed, the price of the portable device itself.

Type II and III PCMCIA cards can contain communication devices such as fax/modems, infrared transceivers, wireless radios, pagers, and small computer systems interface (SCSI) adapters that enable you to connect your portable to peripheral hardware such as a CD-ROM drive. Type III PCMCIA cards, which are thicker than types I and II, actually contain small hard drives and tend to cost less per Mb, but they consume more power. Computers that have a type III PCMCIA slot can accept either a type III PCMCIA card or two type I- or type II-sized cards. Most of the newer portable computers are being manufactured with built-in type II or III slots.

Pocket or Palmtop Computers

HP 200 LX Palmtop PC

The archetype of large-capacity pocket computers is probably the Hewlett Packard (HP) 200 LX (Figure 10-1). This unit, which measures 3.4 × 6.3 inches × 1 inch thick and weighs 11 ounces, is at the upper limit of size and weight to be a comfortable pocket computing companion. The basic unit is essentially an IBM-XT–generation computer using DOS. Although the processor is slow by today's standards, the unit is more than adequate for collecting and maintaining a large amount of information in a simple nonrelational database or spreadsheet format. The unit runs for several weeks on two AA alkaline batteries.

The device offers a choice of two internal memory configurations: 1 Mb or 2 Mb. This "onboard" memory can be configured with up to about 640 Kb dedicated to running system software, and the remaining memory (up to 1360 Kb for the 2-Mb model) is available for storage of your data. Capacity can be enhanced by the addition of a PCMCIA card. The HP 200 LX has a slot to accept one PCMCIA type II card. In contrast to the memory cards supplied by Psion or Sharp (discussed in following sections), no battery is required for the HP 200 LX to maintain the data when these cards are removed from the unit.

Since the unit is IBM-compatible, you have access to a lot of software, at least in theory. In practical terms, the small screen, CGA display (older technology), and inability to access extended memory produce some limitations. The 5-inch diagonal screen can display 80 characters across by 24 lines down. The type size is small for average, middle-aged eyes, so most of the time you will probably want to wear your reading glasses or work with the display toggled to the 64 by 18 or 40 by 16 column-by-row screen. If your DOS software works with the zoom feature or if your vision is excellent, or both, then available programs may fit your needs.

The built-in software accommodates most needs of the average user. The appointment scheduler is very good, the to-do list function is adequate, and the telephone book is excellent. Users can define simple

Figure 10-1. A hand-held portable computer (HP 200 LX Palmtop PC).

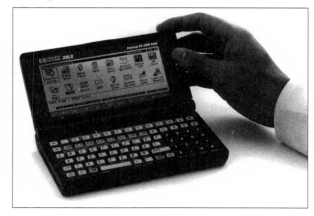

databases for specialized information with a practical limit of about 2000 records. As database size increases, the time required for the unit to process changes increases, and at the extreme, processing a change may require minutes rather than seconds. On the other hand, reference databases that are rarely modified, such as a list of patient names and addresses, can be rapidly accessed even when it is larger than 2000 records. Text files of more than 100 000 characters can be created and edited, and an outline function is included. In addition, documents can be formatted for printing with a popular, albeit limited, group of printers.

In addition to the HP's powerful built-in calculator, the unit includes the Lotus 1-2-3 spreadsheet program. An electronic-mail networking product, Microsoft ccMAIL, is also built in. Finally, a "pocket" version of Quicken, arguably the premier PC personal-finance management software, is built into the computer's permanent memory.

Hewlett Packard provides an excellent "overnight" warranty. If a defect appears, you give HP a credit card number, and they mail you a replacement unit and cancel the charge when the original unit arrives back at HP. Telephone support is available and helpful, but not toll-free. Modem and fax support can be obtained from third-party vendors.

Psion 3a

Less robust in terms of total storage capacity, the Psion 3a is perceptibly thinner, better contoured for a jacket pocket, and slightly easier on the pocketbook. The screen is perhaps the easiest to read of the pocket computers. You can toggle from a display of 40 characters by 9 lines to a full 80 characters by 17 lines. The user interface is graphic and employs a Windows-like menu system, which becomes intuitive and very easy to use with a little practice. Built-in features include a Lotus-like spreadsheet with excellent list-management capabilities (but no macro capability), a memo editor with on-screen formatting, a simple database, an excellent schedule and to-do manager, and a useful calculator.

Out of the box, the Psion 3a gives the user 512 Kb of available memory (similar to the HP 100 LX with the 1-Mb option). The unit has two slots for memory cards. The memory cards are proprietary and of two types: flash and RAM. Flash cards can contain up to 4 Mb of data with no available compression software to double this. Flash cards can be written to once and must be reformatted for the space to become available for reuse. Thus, they are suitable for programs and databases used for reference rather than modification. RAM cards are limited to a maximum of 1 Mb but can be freely written to and read, similar to a hard drive on a standard computer. Each requires its own small battery to maintain information when the card is removed from the machine.

Probably the most convenient feature of the Psion 3a is multitasking, which allows you to have several spreadsheets, one or more memos, and one or more databases all active at the same time. You can then switch from one to another with a few keystrokes without waiting for the programs to save and reload. In contrast, the HP 200 LX requires that one type of application be closed before another of the same type can be opened; with very large files, waiting may require 20 seconds or more, which can be distracting if others are waiting while you fumble with your computing companion.

The Psion also offers a small fax/modem which permits you to send fully formatted text faxes with full support of the built-in word processor. Further, the Psion has a built-in programming language that is actively supported by participants of the Psion section of the CompuServe Palmtop Forum. Interested physicians who can program in BASIC should have no difficulty designing and implementing simple to moderately complex routines that can further customize the Psion to their needs.

Franklin Digital Book System

For beginners in portable computing who want to spend less money and time getting up to speed, another alternative is the Franklin Digital Book (Figure 10-2), a small computerized device that can read and search proprietary ROM cards containing "digital books." The Franklin line of individual titles includes Physicians' Desk Reference, Washington University Manual of Medical Therapeutics, Harrison's Principles of Internal Medicine, Medical Letter Handbook of Adverse Drug Interactions, and Pediatric Handbook. The cost of the Digital Book reader, about $130, is a fraction of that of the palmtops and the Newton (*see under* Newton Message Pad); individual titles are priced at about $100 each.

The catch: The Digital Book is a single-purpose tool that can read only titles produced by Franklin. Users cannot enter any notes on the information (as is possible with other palmtops) or copy informa-

Figure 10-2. A hand-held portable computer (Franklin Digital Book system).

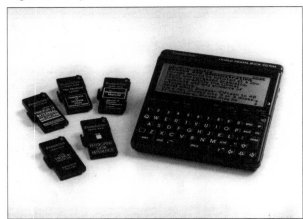

tion from the files and paste it into another document. The Digital Book can store information on a special card provided by Franklin, but this function is inferior to that on other pocket devices. If you want only a portable, solid source of medical information, then the Franklin Digital Book can be a practical alternative.

Wizard Organizer

Sharp Electronics' Wizard Organizers occupy the boundary between electronic organizers and conventional computers. They provide useful time- and expense-recording functions with simple memo, outlining, and calculator functionality. They can interact with the PC and Apple computing environments through their capability of exchanging data with personal computers. The data storage limits of 64 Kb, 256 Kb, and, maximally, about 512 Kb restrict their utility to deal with large amounts of information. Although the units are not programmable by the average user, commercially available programmed cards can be inserted by the user. Some Nikon cameras, for instance, can interface with the Sharp 9600 series to permit the Organizer to memorize and control complex exposure and shutter settings. In the medical arena, Sharp-compatible software is available for purposes such as tracking surgical resident operative experience and results.

Within these limitations, Sharp produces two series, the 9600 and 9500, that provide the user with the ability to record electronic "ink": Simple drawings can be created and stored for later reference. The practical value to medical users might be in creating illustrations for bedside patient education; for example, a cardiologist might create diagrams of procedural findings such as coronary anatomy. In addition, the Sharp 9520FX has a built-in capability to fax information by using an optional, portable fax/modem.

Personal Digital Assistants or Pen-compatible Computers

An intermediate-sized portable computer is too large to fit comfortably into a shirt pocket but is easily held in one hand while using the other to enter data, usually with a pen. The classic examples of PDAs are the Newton Message Pad and the Tandy (Radio Shack) Zoomer.

Newton Message Pad

The first Newton received negative reviews because of limitations with handwriting recognition, user-available memory, software, and battery life. The upgraded Newton Message Pad 110 is more robust (Figure 10-3). Changes include increase of user memory to 1 Mb, ability to defer handwriting recognition in order to simplify use, and price reduction by about $100. Features include simple database functions for scheduling, telephone book management, and simple note entry. Freehand drawing is also available. Capabilities for wireless communication are built in, and nationwide communication support is available via E-World from Apple Computer.

Initially, few medically oriented software programs were available for the Newton. However, increasing attention has been given to the medical uses of this device, and clinically useful products such as

Figure 10-3. The Apple Newton Message Pad 110.

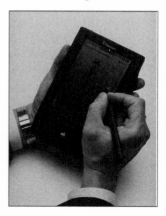

UpToDate (a medical reference resource) and others are beginning to appear. Graffiti, a new handwriting recognition program, promises to strongly enhance the utility of the Newton as well as other pen-based computers for use in medical applications.

Tandy Zoomer

The Zoomer is a palmtop digital assistant designed for pen-enabled data entry with a more conservative approach to handwriting recognition. Individual letters rather than words are accepted, and the initial user success is probably better. The unit is fairly slow, but some of the built-in software may be more helpful than that provided with the Newton. A pen-aware version of the personal-finance program Quicken is built into the Zoomer.

Other Pen Pals

Other Windows-based, pen-enabled computers are also on the market. Some, like the Toshiba Dynapad T200CS or Dauphine DTR-1, are fully functional, sophisticated devices with detachable keyboards and much more weight. This market is growing, and new devices are appearing almost monthly. Recently, a trade magazine, *Pen Computing*, has appeared, and the interested reader might seek additional information there. (*See* the Appendix for more information resources.)

Subnotebooks

As noted earlier, the subnotebooks are the ultra-lightweight derivatives of the full-keyboard "note-book" computers, themselves the laptop progeny designed for briefcase portability. The subnotebooks are one of the most rapidly growing markets in personal computing, and, when little is lost in terms of processor speed, hard-disk size, and screen readability, smaller indeed appears to be better. Figure 10-4 shows a subnotebook computer.

If you choose to buy a subnotebook, consideration should be given to weight, battery life, processor speed, RAM, hard-disk capacity, and display readability. Many of these units require external floppy drives, which may become a comparison issue. Special attention should be paid to the topic of battery technology and battery-charging options.

New battery technology, including nickel-metal-hydride (NMHi), lithium-ion (Li Ion), and air-lithium batteries, is replacing the current nickel-cadmium technology. The major new benefits are more charge

Figure 10-4. A subnotebook computer with the PCMCIA card partially ejected.

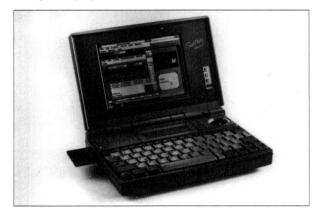

capacity per unit weight and freedom from "battery memory." The memory phenomenon with nickel-cadmium batteries requires the batteries to be completely discharged on a regular basis for optimal performance. When you do not need to worry about fully discharging a battery before recharging it again, having the computer as a constant companion becomes easier.

When choosing a lightweight computing companion, look at the battery-charging hardware. It makes little sense to pay a lot for portable technology and then receive an AC adapter that weighs as much as the computer. An unusually innovative approach by IBM is having batteries that can be plugged directly into an AC outlet for recharging. The time required for battery recharging should be less than 3 hours, or you will sacrifice portability simply because the battery is not recharged when you are ready to go. The Hewlett Packard Omni series brings battery charge up to a useful amount (70% to 80%) within 1 hour and then trickles up to a full charge during an additional 1 to 2 hours.

Manufacturers' and reviewers' estimates of battery life can be ambiguous. If a device uses a PCMCIA storage device, the battery life may be twice that of an identical configuration using hard-disk storage. Devices that use both hard drives and PCMCIA cards have a useful battery life somewhere in between. Also consider the tradeoff between battery life and unit weight. If the unit weighs 3 pounds and carries a 6-ounce battery that lasts 4 hours, is it less portable than a 4.5-pound unit with a 1.5-pound battery that lasts 8 hours? The lighter unit plus an extra battery weighs less than the heavier unit and lasts just as long.

HP Omni 530

The Omni 300, a 386 subnotebook computer—featuring instant on/off, RAM-resident versions of Microsoft Word and Excel, PCMCIA solid-state data storage, and 8 hours of battery life—was a computing breakthrough. The use of advanced power management features, a metal hydride battery, a passive matrix liquid-crystal display (LCD) screen, and PCMCIA solid-state technology enabled the creation of a powerful computer that was small and light enough to be used as a truly portable companion. When the Omni 300 was introduced, most competing products weighed more than 6 pounds and had a practical battery life of less than 3 hours.

Within a year of its introduction, the Omni 300 was replaced by a similar unit with a 486/25-MHz processor. The current Omni is the 530 (2.9 pounds) with a 130-Mb hard drive, 4 Mb of RAM (expandable to 12 Mb), and a 33-MHz processor with two type-II PCMCIA slots. Using compression software, the HP Omni 530 has a potential storage capacity of 420 Mb in an ultra-lightweight box that features a full-sized keyboard, relatively fast processing speed, and enough RAM to run several major Windows applications at the same time. Indeed, the Omni 530 is soon to be replaced by the 600c that weighs 3.9 pounds, has a 3- to 3.5-hour battery life, and features a passive matrix color screen.

The major shortcoming of the current Omni is its lack of a color, or even a backlighted, screen. In spite of this, industry reviewers still give high marks to the Omni for its major values: high portability, immediate on/off access to major software productivity tools, useful battery life, and an excellent keyboard.

Shortcomings such as the reflective screen are the price paid for an extra hour or two of usability before the battery needs changing. An extra battery weighs a pocketable 6 ounces.

Keeping Up with 3-Pound Subnotebooks

This area of portable computing is rapidly changing and expanding in both the PC and Macintosh environments. Popular computer magazines regularly update and compare the latest entrants into this arena. Consulting such resources will give you a clearer picture of the available products and the state-of-the-art key features such as battery life, memory, storage, screen readability, and cost.

HOW CAN I SUCCESSFULLY IMPLEMENT PORTABLE COMPUTING TECHNOLOGY IN MY PRACTICE?

Should you consider implementing portable computing technology in your practice? Definitely. The cost of portable devices has dropped, and their functionality has increased to the point where many physicians will find it attractive to implement these tools. Many clinicians are already using portable computers and imagining how difficult it would be to function well without them.

Getting Ready To Go Portable

Before you take the plunge, make two lists. The first is the list of databases you wish to carry and use. The most obvious kinds are appointments, telephone numbers, to-do lists, and patient information. Additional possibilities include treatment guidelines, drug information, selected medical abstracts, other medical databases, and personal financial records. The larger your list of databases, the more important is the amount of memory for data storage. If the average number of characters for a telephone-book entry is 250, a telephone book of 1000 entries will require 250 000 characters, the limit for a 256-Kb pocket device. If manipulating free-form text is important for such things as drug information or medical databases, the built-in software must be flexible enough to handle this, or the device must support third-party text management software.

The second list is that of the tasks you want to perform. Again, the most obvious tasks are maintaining a few simple lists and an appointment schedule. Additional possibilities include automated generation of consultation and procedural reports that can be faxed to referring physicians' offices and elsewhere, maintenance of text databases, and utilization of specific medical software. Again, the more elaborate your requirements, the larger is the device you are likely to require. Try to keep sight of the fact that you are choosing a portable companion, not a desktop substitute.

Finally, you should consider the logistics of using a portable device. Each of us has a self-image that may not include porting a subnotebook on rounds and opening it for use during committee meetings. Some may not even be comfortable with a perceptible bulge in their jacket pocket. So when you consider buying a portable computer, candidly assess your comfort in transporting the device wherever you go and using it in the presence of your patients and colleagues.

Selecting a Portable Computer

Pocket or Palmtop Computers

If at all possible, go to retail outlets such as Circuit City or Service Merchandise and look at several units. See how they actually feel in your pocket. Look at the appointment and to-do functions. These should appear pleasing and intuitive to you. Available user memory should be at least 256 Kb. A spreadsheet is excellent for maintaining simple lists and should be included in the initial purchase. A spreadsheet is built into the Psion and HP hand-held units but must be purchased as a separate card with the Sharp. Call the manufacturer of selected units and ask for information packets. Browse through the manuals while at the store.

Spend 5 to 10 minutes typing something meaningful on the keyboard. The palmtops are not meant for long periods of typing, but on an airplane or during other unproductive times, you may want to prepare memos or outline a paper. On the run, you will discover "thumb typing." This feat is accomplished by holding the unit in both palms and using your thumbs to hit the keys. The feel of the unit may go a long way in helping you decide what you want.

Select the brand that best combines the features you like, the size that you will feel comfortable carrying daily, and the price you are willing to invest.

The major advantage to the HP palmtop is its industry-standard conservatism. The 200 LX uses standard PCMCIA cards, runs a large number of standard DOS applications, has extensive third-party support, and has a prodigious storage capacity. The *Palmtop Paper,* an excellent bimonthly publication that supports HP palmtop computing, featured medical uses of the HP LX series in a recent issue (*see* Appendix, Chapter 10). Medical software was listed, including pharmaceutical and drug interaction databases, a patient history-taking assistant, and the Quick Medical Reference diagnostic decision support program. An initial choice might be the 2-Mb configuration, which leaves you more than enough data-storage space (1.3 Mb) to get started before you need to add additional memory.

The Psion 3a enjoys an enthusiastic support forum (Go Palmtop) on CompuServe and probably has more units purchased than the HP, although it lacks the HP's third-party software support. The Psion is fun and easy to use but utilizes a nonstandard storage card. Additional memory should be included in the initial purchase plan if extensive use is contemplated.

PDAs or Pen-enabled Portable Companions

Devices such as the Newton Message Pad, Compaq Concierto, IBM ThinkPad 700C, and Fujitsu 500C incorporate pen software and range in size from a palmtop to a laptop. Pen-enabled computing technology is so new and continually changing that any detailed discussion is soon obsolete. Get up-to-date information from your retail electronics dealer. (*See,* in addition, the information resources listed in the Appendix.)

As noted earlier in this chapter, the Newton is beginning to receive considerable attention in the medical community. A useful collection of products is now available, and many others are under development. In addition, the Newton provides a lot of functionality per unit weight. Many believe that the Apple Newton technology is, indeed, the future of portable computing and communication.

Subnotebooks

Many 486-class subnotebooks weigh less than 4.5 pounds, and a subset of this type of computer weighs less than 3.5 pounds. Of the latter, the HP Omni 530 is probably closest to the benchmark portable companion. Less than 3 pounds and with a useful battery life of about 4 hours, the Omni lacks a backlighted screen but is exceptionally easy to carry. It is worth reiterating that this device features instant on/off, instant switching between applications, an excellent keyboard, and the largest screen of the PC subnotebooks. Gateway also manufactures a subnotebook in the 3-pound weight class. The Gateway 2000 Handbook seems to be a solid choice except for its shorter battery life and some compromises with the display and keyboard. The entry-level Compaq Aero, weighing in at 3.5 pounds, has also received favorable reviews.

If you are committed to carrying more weight, the Toshiba Portégé, IBM ThinkPad 510, and Zenith Z-Lite 425L, Model 170W, subnotebooks have received

good reviews. Apple also manufactures a subnotebook weighing less than 4.5 pounds.

Note that the available products and features will probably change considerably between the writing and reading of this book. You are strongly encouraged to consult popular computer magazines and other resources to assess the state of the art if you are considering buying a portable device. Of course, you should also consider the types of software you intend to use when deciding about which portable device(s) best meets your needs.

Deciding on Software

Subnotebooks

If you are a computer novice, you should look at computer magazines for information about general-purpose software. Decide whether you want to use word processing, spreadsheet, database, and faxing programs (*see* Chapter 11), and discuss these with your colleagues and knowledgeable salespeople.

With my HP Omni 530 subnotebook computer, I use Microsoft Word for Windows 6.0 and Excel 5.0 as my word processor and spreadsheet, respectively. I use Commence as my textual database and personal-information manager and WinFax Pro 4.0 for faxes. An alternative personal-information manager that many use is Ecco, which features an outline function but does not hold as much textual information as Commence. For database records, Microsoft Access runs well on the Omni but does not do well if the database is stored on a PCMCIA card because it does not seem to recognize the automatic power-off.

As for available medical software, the subnotebooks are, of course, full-fledged computers that can generally use any of the clinical programs discussed in this book.

Palmtops and PDAs

Various medical products have been created or adapted for the hand-held devices. We have noted the dedicated titles for the Franklin Digital Books: PDR, Harrison's Principles of Internal Medicine, The Medical Letter Handbook of Adverse Drug Reactions, The Merck Manual, and others. A medical program called Hippocrates for the Newton allows physicians to organize patient schedules, hospital rounds, prescriptions, and on-call care using the unit; information can be loaded to and from desktop computers (*see under* Transferring Your Files), and prescriptions can be faxed to pharmacies using the Newton's communication capabilities. As mentioned earlier, UpToDate and other useful clinical references are also available for the Newton, and many others are being developed. Available for the HP palmtop are several medical programs, including a continuing medical education documenter and a diagnostic decision support program, among others. (*See* the Appendix for more sources of information about these and other medical programs for the palmtops and PDAs.)

Creating Your First Data Files

This section offers some specific suggestions for getting started with the multifaceted task of organizing your personal and professional information and for developing the habit of carrying and consulting your portable computing device.

Create a database called "phonebook" and one called "info." Make sure the info database has a title, subtitle, and note field. Create two spreadsheets with names like "mileage" and "expenses." For the mileage spreadsheet, create columns for the date, odometer reading, and trips. For the expenses spreadsheet, create columns for the date, paid to, paid for, paid with, and the amount. You may, of course, use any field and column names you wish, but start with as few as possible.

Create a spreadsheet (or database) called "patients." Next, create a column (or field) for the date, name, and details. Keep it simple at first. If you want to track the time spent with patients, include columns labeled "start" and "end." For billing, you might want a field for CPT (Current Procedural Terminology) codes. Create a memo file named "scratch." Use this for scribbling miscellaneous items as they arise during the day.

Spend an evening creating a set-up similar to that suggested above, and add all of your recurrent staff and hospital meetings to the calendar. Birthdays and anniversaries can also be entered. Put some important personal and professional telephone numbers into your "phonebook," using a consistent "Last name, First name" format for the name field. In the to-do section of the scheduler, enter some of your activities for the next week. Include a category for telephone calls to make, personal items, hospital-related tasks, and tasks to be delegated to someone else. Priorities might be assigned according to the Covey system: 1=important and urgent; 2=important and not urgent; 3 = unimportant and urgent; and 4 = unimportant and not urgent.

Agree with your nurse or secretary that, when you forget a meeting or appointment that is "in the computer," it is your fault. Otherwise, it is the assistant's fault. This method encourages your assistants' full-hearted support.

Pick a morning you feel unusually compulsive and begin by entering your odometer reading before you start to work. List short, one- or two-letter codes for each of yesterday's trips. For the next 2 to 3 months, keep the device with you wherever you go. On rounds, as you see each patient, enter the date, name, and a short comment. At the office, have your nurse or secretary copy billing information and update your appointment schedule; then continue to make a short entry for each patient you see.

Any time you have to look up a telephone number, add it to your "phonebook" database. At staff meetings, when announcements are made of new services, new requirements for documentation, or new third-party reviewers, make an appropriate name and number entry in your phonebook. When you open mail, add interesting continuing medical education and product announcements. During the day, when you want to scribble a quick reminder, use the "scratch" file. When you make a commitment or promise, note it in the to-do section of your appointment book. When you need some information you remember having previously entered, look it up in your personal assistant.

Do things as compulsively as possible for several weeks, and then reassess the situation. Eliminate or change any categories to better suit your needs, and add anything you think might be helpful. Continue using the device for another month or two. By the end of that time, you will discover either that you are forgetting to take the portable device with you each morning or that you are finding it indispensable. Either way, you will have discovered whether it is helpful enough to carry around and use.

Transferring Your Files

An important tactical consideration is the transfer of material from your portable device to and from your desktop unit. The ability to transfer files is surely a benchmark of the portability of the data.

Transfer of files between pocket computers and desktop units is fairly straightforward, but translation of content from a pocket unit's data structure to standard PC software often is not. The information contained within the HP, Psion, Sharp, and other hand-held devices is stored in proprietary format. Even after transferring files to a PC or Macintosh computer, you may not be able to read them using standard third-party software. In this case, you need conversion software.

Each of these companies sells software and cables to transfer data to personal computers, but the functionality and sophistication vary. Even when a manufacturer sells a data import-export product, the software may not perform as well as the user legitimately expects. New hardware is commonly released months before the software and cables, which are needed for linking to personal computers; and the functionality of this connectivity software seems to reflect a relatively low commercial priority.

Hewlett Packard, Psion, Apple, and Sharp each sell software and cables suitable for transferring files and information to and from a PC or Macintosh for backup. In each case, software is available to convert the information contained in the palmtop to a format that is understood by commercial software packages. But none of the available data-exchange software is flawless, and you will have to commit some time and effort before such transfer becomes second nature.

Hardware Support for Data Transfer

The classic means of exchanging information between computers is by a cable connecting the serial ports of two devices. Such cables are generally available for all of the computers discussed above. Newer technology such as infrared signals is available for data transfer, for example, between HP palmtops, between HP palmtops and HP Omni, and between Sharp Organizers and various printers.

PCMCIA cards can also be a practical way to transfer data (or even devices such as a fax/modem) between desktop and portable computers. In many cases, this strategy is preferred. To be successful, you must make sure that your portable and desktop computers have compatible slots (for example, both type II) and that each device can utilize the capabilities of the PCMCIA card you intend to transfer. Equipped with a modem, your portable device can serve as a window to a wide array of medical information and communications resources.

Many hospitals provide free or nominally priced access to medical, pharmacy, and toxicology databases via telephone lines. (*See* Chapter 8 for additional information on commercial databases and other resources accessible online.) In addition, wireless telecommunications capabilities are beginning to appear in portable devices and will enhance the ease of information transfer. If online or fax functionality sounds attractive to you, then you should investigate all the communication hardware options for each portable device you are considering.

Putting the Portable to Work: A Personal Approach

About 10 years ago, I began using the MEDLINE database available through Knowledge Index, an off-hours service now available via CompuServe. Each month I downloaded 200 to 300 abstracts covering selected cardiology journals and cardiology articles from internal medicine journals. I am now using a Word for Windows macro to "read" these articles, strip out extraneous text, and save the result in a format that can be imported into a Commence database. As I review these abstracts using an HP Omni 600C, often between patient visits or when at home, I fax a list of needed printouts to my secretary and generally have copies the next afternoon.

Commence is also used to keep a list of patient demographics and a linked list of very brief patient visit and procedure notes that are entered as they occur. Quarterly, the business office creates a diskette of the names and addresses of patients to update my portable database. When called about a patient problem on the weekend or evening, I can refer to these useful data.

I write several medical newsletter-type reviews and keep these on the Omni, to be worked on using Word, whenever and wherever time permits. When an article is completed, I fax it to the appropriate institution. Word also has a powerful forms feature that permits me to create procedure report templates that I can complete and print (using fax printers at area hospitals) as quickly as they might have been dictated.

I use the Lotus 1-2-3 application on an HP 100 LX to keep spreadsheets of odometer readings and trips for tax purposes, records of deductible or reimbursable expenses, billable time spent reviewing medical records for third parties or attorneys, and the titles and performers of my music collection on compact disc. Several Lotus 1-2-3 macros that I wrote simplify data entry. Tax and reimbursable expense information is transferred to an Excel spreadsheet on the Omni from which reports are printed. Finally, I use the HP hand-held device to maintain a telephone-book database and manage my schedule exactly as I outlined in the section Creating Your First Data Files.

In the past, I have used PowerPoint and Excel on a desktop computer to create lectures for students and residents; I then sent these files to our medical illustration department via CompuServe for slide creation. In the future, I plan to use the Omni's external monitor port and a computer-enabled overhead projector to present these lectures, which will eliminate the cost and inconvenience of making slides and make it much easier to change the lecture on Monday and use the new material on Tuesday. Another future project is to use the Omni to take advantage of Physicians' Online's free access to the Physicians' GenRx database of pharmaceutical monographs and other medical databases. I also hope to create a personalized cardiovascular information database that can be put on the HP 100/200 LX for use by the residents that rotate on my service.

The rapid advances in wireless technology, combined with increasingly sophisticated portable and online systems, will make portable computing devices an indispensable information management tool for a growing number of physicians. Now is an excellent time to begin exploring the usefulness of these resources.

11

COMPUTER BASICS

Karin Rex

If you are a computer novice, this chapter will give you the basic information necessary to make a sound decision when buying a computer. The section titled Bits, Bytes, and Other Buzzwords is an introduction to computer jargon. Having a solid grasp of computer "technobabble" should help to make buying a computer less intimidating. Buying Hardware is a primer for picking a computer platform (for example, a PC or a Macintosh computer), choosing components for a computer system, and knowing how to shop. Understanding Software guides you through the popular types of computer programs and offers some tips on the conventions of software usage.

If you are already experienced in the computer world, then you can use this chapter as a general refresher or basic reference source. Whether or not you are experienced with computers, this material will provide some context and perspective for much of the information presented in the other chapters. To round out this introduction to computer basics and help ensure that this book works for you, a glossary of important technical terms follows this chapter.

Bits, Bytes, and Other Buzzwords

When you buy a computer, you can easily be overwhelmed by the many numbers and technical terms involved. It is intimidating to walk into a computer store unprepared and come face-to-face with a question-spouting salesperson (who most likely works on commission and sees dollar signs painted across your puzzled brow). Even reading computer advertisements can be frustrating if you do not comprehend the jargon and numbers. Although you can hire a consultant to advise you, being able to converse intelligently about your specific computing needs and understand what you are buying is the best course.

Units of Measurement

First, you must understand how computing power and storage capacity are measured in a computer. Some of the first questions a computer salesperson will probably ask you are about this subject. What size hard disk do you want? How much RAM do you think you will need? (If the first question is "How much do you want to spend?" leave immediately.)

A *bit* is the smallest unit of information that a computer can work with. A bit is represented by the binary digits 1 and 0, which, like the poles of a light switch, represent "on" and "off"; to the computer, information is processed as sequences of on-and-off voltage pulsations. Bits are combined into larger groups that the computer processes as a unit. A *byte* is the basic unit and is composed of 8 bits. Translated into a more tangible measurement, 1 byte can represent a single character (such as the letter "a" or the numeral "4"). For efficiency, bytes are grouped together as kilobytes, megabytes, and gigabytes.

A *kilobyte* (abbreviated Kb and often called a "K") is frequently used to measure file size and is equal to 1024 bytes. A *megabyte* (abbreviated Mb and often called a "meg")—often used to measure memory, hard-disk space, and file size—is equal to 1024 kilobytes. A *gigabyte* (abbreviated Gb and often called a "gig") is usually used to measure hard-disk space and very large files and is equal to 1024 megabytes.

Most of the numbers you have to understand when buying a computer concern *memory* and *hard-disk storage*.

Memory

Like humans, a computer needs short-term, or working, memory to process information. Working memory in a computer is called RAM (random-access memory). When power is cut to a computer, everything in the short-term memory is erased. This loss of information does not apply to saved files, which are recorded in a separate, long-term storage area.

You may think of memory in terms of working space—similar to desk space. If an architect has a small desk, she or he has difficulty spreading large blueprints on it. If the desk is large, the blueprints can be spread out easily and worked on comfortably. Computer memory is like desk space. More computer memory means the computer has more space to process information. If your computer has only a small amount of RAM (2 or 4 Mb), you will probably be confined to using one application at a time. If your computer has a large amount of RAM (8 or more Mb), then you can often work on several applications at once or work with certain kinds of graphic files and other applications that require substantial memory.

ROM, or read-only memory, is another type of computer memory. Vital information is programmed permanently into a computer's ROM at the factory and cannot be altered. Just as with the CD-ROM products described in Chapter 9, you can read the information, but generally you cannot write to the disk. ROM is used to store programs (called firmware) that give a computer instructions for essential tasks. You do not need to worry about ROM, as you have no control over it.

Some people confuse working memory with storage. Remember that RAM is temporary. To permanently store files and programs, you need storage space—namely, a hard disk—and its capacity has nothing to do with how much RAM your computer has.

Storage Space

A *hard disk* is usually housed inside the CPU (central processing unit) box. Think of a hard disk as an electronic filing cabinet. The hard disk stores your operating-system software, application software, and data files. The bigger the hard disk, the more you can store on it, and the more it will cost—similar to the difference between buying a two-drawer or a five-drawer filing cabinet.

Hard disks come in many sizes, ranging from 20 Mb to over 1 Gb. The larger the hard disk, the cheaper the per-megabyte cost for storage. A word of advice: Never skimp on hard-disk space—you will regret it all too soon. Some of the more sophisticated and graphic-intensive programs discussed in this book require a lot of storage space. Keep in mind, however, that you can always upgrade to a larger hard disk later or add an external hard disk for additional storage. An external hard disk is a separate unit from the CPU.

Hardware and Software

When you buy a computer, you are usually concerned with hardware first. Hardware is any physical piece of computer-system equipment, for example, a monitor, keyboard, mouse, or printer. You should, however, have an understanding of the types of software you want to use before you buy the hardware—a specific program may only run on a specific type of hardware. The main distinction in hardware is that between the Macintosh and the PC (*see under* Buying Hardware).

Software is made up of coded instructions that may be stored on a CD-ROM, a diskette, or your computer's hard disk; software determines what you can do with your computer. The two types of software are *application* and *operating system*. An example of application software is a program such as ClinicaLogic, which allows you to use your computer to create and manage electronic medical records. The clinical information management programs discussed in this book are application software. Several popular general-purpose application software programs are discussed later in this chapter.

An operating system (also known as an OS; pronounced "oh-es") is the master-control software that runs a computer. This software is automatically started whenever a computer is turned on, and it stays running the entire time that the computer is on. An example of operating system software is DOS 6.x, which is the sixth generation of the *disk operating system* (DOS) software created by Microsoft Corporation. The Macintosh operating system software is currently called System 7.x. (The "x" stands for a digit denoting upgrade versions released between major revisions of the software.)

Application software is written to work specifically with one type of operating system software. A program created for one operating system generally does not work on a different operating system. For example, you cannot use the Macintosh version of the diagnostic decision support program Quick Medical Reference (QMR) on a computer whose operating system is DOS.

The Macintosh system software comes loaded on the computer when you buy it and is included in the price. If you buy an IBM or IBM clone, DOS is usually loaded on the computer and also included in the price. However, DOS requires memorization and typing of commands and is not considered an easy operating system to use.

An alternative to DOS is the Microsoft Windows environment, a popular choice among many PC users for a working interface. Windows, an extension to DOS, was created by Microsoft Corporation for PCs. Unlike DOS itself, Windows uses a *graphical user interface* (GUI; pronounced "gooey") and is considered easier to use. The GUI allows you to communicate with your computer by selecting icons (pictures) and menu items, using a pointing device such as a mouse instead of typing memorized commands as with DOS. To run Windows on your computer, however, you must use DOS as the background operating system.

Networks

If you are buying more than one computer or adding to an already computerized environment, you should also understand the term *network*. A network is a system of connections that enables one computer to "talk" to another computer or to another piece of peripheral equipment such as a printer. The method of connection may be as simple as a single cable connecting two computers in the same room (known as a local area network, or LAN) or as complex as a system that connects computers all over the world using telephone lines or other specialized cables (known as a wide area network, or WAN).

On its simplest level, the purpose of a network is the easy exchange of information. For example, in a large medical center, it may be easier and more efficient for a diagnostic laboratory in one location to send a report electronically through the network to physicians in other locations than to physically transport the information on paper (especially if such transmittals occur frequently throughout the day). In many offices, hospitals, and medical centers, large or small, the importance of exchanging clinical and other data is leading to installation of both LANs and WANs.

The use of networks for e-mail, access to information databases, discussion forums, and other functions of value to the practitioner is discussed at length in Chapter 8.

Multimedia

A commonly used buzzword is *multimedia,* which refers to a dynamic and stimulating format for presenting information. Multimedia material can contain information in various media, including still images, moving video, animation, and sound, in addition to unformatted or formatted text. An *interactive* multimedia presentation allows the user to control the flow and content of a presentation by selecting items on the screen or typing answers to questions. This technology can be particularly useful in patient education and continuing medical education applications.

Viewing multimedia material, however, requires a powerful computer system. You need an abundance of both memory and hard-disk storage space as well as sound capabilities and special video software. In addition, a CD-ROM player is usually required, as the vast storage capacity of a CD-ROM is usually needed to contain the large multimedia data files. Existing computer systems can be upgraded to run multimedia applications. Alternatively, multimedia-capable personal computers, called MPCs, with all the requirements built in, are available for purchase.

Buying Hardware

As I suggested earlier, when you buy a computer, you should pick a *platform* first. A platform is a type of computer environment. The two most popular types of personal computer platforms are Apple Macintoshes (called Macs) and IBM-type computers (called PCs). PC is an abbreviation for personal computer. Although a Macintosh is certainly considered a personal computer, this abbreviation is normally used to indicate a non-Macintosh computer such as an IBM-compatible personal computer.

A third type of platform is a specialized network environment such as UNIX. This environment typically requires a special operating system and hardware and software. Since the UNIX environment is so well suited to network applications, practice management systems often use it. However, this chapter focuses on the Macintosh and PC platforms, and most of the applications discussed in the other chapters run on one or both of these platforms.

Macintosh versus PC

IBM makes PCs, but so do dozens of other manufacturers. When a PC is made by a company other than IBM, it is called a *clone* or an *IBM-compatible*. When properly selected, IBM-compatibles offer excellent performance and value; in fact, some of the best PCs are those made by companies other than IBM. Because many different companies manufacture PCs,

pricing is generally competitive. Until recently, only Apple made computers that could run Macintosh software. However, Mac clones are now becoming available.

Macintoshes and PCs are competitive in regard to price, although this was not always true. For the first few years of their existence, Macs were priced much higher than PCs, but today you can find the same power for roughly the same price.

Some people believe that Macs are easier to use than PCs. Although true in some cases, this judgment is becoming less true with time. If a Mac is compared with a PC using DOS, then it is safe to say that the Mac is much easier to use. If, however, a Mac is compared with a PC running Windows, the ease-of-use argument for a Macintosh fades. Both the Macintosh and Windows environments are relatively easy to use.

If you need a computer for intensive imaging or graphic presentation purposes, the Macintosh is probably the machine of choice. The reason may be as straightforward as the wide array of graphic arts software available for the Mac or as abstract as the "feel" of the Mac or the strength of its reputation in the graphic arts community. I cannot overemphasize, however, that you should have a good idea of what programs you plan to use before deciding on your computer platform. When you get excited about new software, learn whether it runs on the Mac or PC; many, but not all, of the programs noted in this book are available for both.

If you want to be able to share computer files with a certain group of colleagues, ask what type of computer hardware and software they use. Today, using Mac files on a PC and vice versa is relatively uncomplicated. However, for true ease of use, you may wish to buy hardware and software similar to that of your coworkers. Some of the newer Mac models (called Power Macs) run PC software such as Windows and DOS as well as Macintosh software. Currently, no PCs can run Mac software.

To make an informed decision about selecting a platform, try both types of machine for yourself or at least get a demonstration of each. By understanding your needs, considering the software you will be using, and consulting with your colleagues, you can make a clear choice.

A Basic Computer System

Once you have selected a platform, you can then choose specific hardware components. The most basic computer system includes a central processing unit, monitor, keyboard, printer, and mouse.

Central Processing Unit

The CPU is a tiny chip, or microprocessor, that is the brain of a computer. Traditionally, however, the entire box housing the chip, hard disk, disk drive, and other components is referred to as the CPU. (If you picture a typical computer, the CPU box would be the main unit to which the keyboard and monitor are attached.)

Speed of information processing is an important consideration when selecting a CPU. The speed of a CPU is determined by two factors: the number of bits it can process at one time and the clock speed. The more bits a computer can process in one chunk, the faster it can finish a calculation. The older PCs, using an 80286 chip, process 16 bits at a time. The newer 80386 and 80486 chips can process 32 bits at a time. Clock speed, which determines how fast a CPU can process information, is measured in megahertz (MHz, millions of cycles per second). A higher number means a faster clock speed and a more expensive computer. Typically, the clock speed is seen in the model number of a computer. For example, if an advertisement offers a 486/33 or a 486/66, the first number refers to the chip (Intel 80486) and the second number, to the clock speed (33 or 66 MHz).

Inside the CPU box are one or two *floppy-disk drives*. A disk drive is necessary to read from and write to a floppy disk. A floppy disk (or diskette) is one device used to transport or back up information. Physically, a floppy disk is a thin, round piece of magnetically coated mylar enclosed in a stiff plastic sheath. The 3.5-inch disk, although it is not flexible, is still by tradition called a floppy disk. A Macintosh uses only this size disk. PCs can use either 3.5- or 5.25-inch disks, or both, depending on the available drives. The 3.5-inch format is currently the most common. You should be aware that many newer computers are also available with CD-ROM drives built into the CPU box (*see under* Computing Peripherals).

Diskettes make it easy to share and transport data. For example, to share a long list of literature citations with another physician, one convenient method is to copy the data onto a diskette and share that. (Such data sharing is most convenient if you and your colleague are using the same platform.) Diskettes are also used to back up data. Data stored on a hard disk are stored permanently—that is, until you choose to erase it. However, hard disks are not infallible. A bad electrical storm or other internal problems could cause a hard disk to "crash," leaving you with a large loss of data. For this reason, you must habitually copy important files from your hard disk onto a floppy disk or other back-up medium to protect your information (*see under* Backing Up Your Data).

Monitor

The monitor is the part of your computer that resembles a television screen. Without a monitor, you cannot see what your computer is doing. To make the CPU and monitor work together, the CPU contains a video display adapter (or "board"). The adapter translates what you do on the keyboard, or with the mouse, into a picture on the screen.

Monitors are classified by adapter type: EGA, CGA, VGA, or Super VGA. The EGA (enhanced graphics adapter) and CGA (color graphics adapter) are two all-but-outmoded monitor types. The CGA was the first adapter to allow graphics on screen; with a CGA, a monitor can display 640×200 pixels in only one color. Offering a much finer image, the VGA (video graphics adapter, or virtual graphics array) monitors display a resolution of 640×480 pixels in 16 colors on the screen. Super VGA is an extension of the standard VGA monitors that expands the screen resolution to 800×600 pixels or to 1024×768 pixels. Super VGA images are noticeably sharper than those of standard VGAs.

Monitors with a Super VGA adapter are the most expensive. Other factors that affect the price of a monitor are refresh rate, resolution, color capability, and, of course, size.

Refresh rate, measured in cycles per second, is the speed at which an image is redrawn on the computer screen. The larger the number, the faster the redraw. Resolution is the number of dots per inch (DPI) that a monitor can show; the higher the DPI, the better the image. One single dot is a pixel, the smallest element that a monitor can display. Each pixel is part of the mosaic of dots that compose the screen image.

Monitors are available in monochrome, grayscale, and color. A monochrome monitor uses only one color on a differently colored background, for example, white on a black background. A grayscale monitor shows a range of gray between black and white. You can expect to pay more money for a monitor that is capable of grayscale. A color monitor is more expensive than either a monochrome or grayscale monitor but is easier on the eye and very popular.

Monitor sizes vary from 9 to 20 inches or more. To choose a monitor, think about the type of work you will be doing. If you will be using a computer infrequently and will only be displaying a relatively small amount of information on the screen, such as with a diagnostic decision support system, then a smaller monitor would probably be sufficient. If, however, you will be looking at large volumes of data for prolonged periods of time, such as with electronic medical records, then you should select a larger screen.

Keyboard

Another piece of hardware you need to choose is a keyboard. Most computers come with a standard 105-key keyboard for information input. This keyboard has a separate set of cursor keys, a numeric keypad, and so-called function keys. Cursor keys (also called arrow keys) are a set of keys used to move the on-screen cursor. A numeric keypad is a set of keys for typing numbers. Function keys are marked F1 through F12 or F15 and can be used as shortcuts to issue commands in most software programs. A keyboard with function keys is not absolutely necessary but is useful and generally worth the extra money.

Some Mac models and most portable computers come with a slightly smaller keyboard that combines the numeric keypad and the cursor keys. Unless you have space constraints, the 105-key keyboard is the most comfortable and useful. Apple makes an adjustable keyboard that is ergonomically designed for comfort; the keyboard splits in the middle, allowing for various finger placements.

Another factor differentiating keyboards is key action, or touch. Some click; some are relatively noiseless. Try before you buy, and choose what feels comfortable.

Mouse

A mouse is a hand-held pointing device that allows you to communicate with your computer. For Macintoshes and PCs running Windows, either of which will likely be your first choice in a platform, a mouse is required. A standard mouse is usually included with a system if you are buying a Macintosh or a PC with Windows; it has a ball on the bottom and one or more buttons on the top. You work the mouse by rolling it on a flat surface such as a desk or mouse pad to position the on-screen pointer.

An alternative to the standard mouse is the trackball-style mouse. A trackball mouse has a large ball positioned on top of the mouse, with buttons on each side. You work a trackball mouse by keeping the mouse stationary and rolling the ball on top to position the on-screen pointer. The trackball-mouse is especially useful if you have little room on your desk and is commonly used in portable computers such as subnotebooks.

For input of information, the mouse and the keyboard are the most common methods. But computers may also be voice-activated or pen-enabled. (*See* Chapter 10 for examples of pen-enabled, portable computing devices that may be of interest to you.)

Printer

Another important piece of computer hardware is the printer. A printer allows you to print out your patient records, literature search results, and other information you have accessed. Unless you think you will not need paper copies of your work (which is generally not the case), or you plan to copy your files to a diskette and take them elsewhere to be printed (an impractical approach in most situations), then you will need a printer. The printer you choose must be compatible with your computer platform. Remember this if you are putting an additional computer on an office network that is already equipped with a printer.

Two factors that affect the price of a printer are image resolution and output speed. The resolution of a printer is measured in dots per inch; the higher the DPI, the better the quality of the printing. Output is measured in pages per minute (PPM), which denotes the speed of page-oriented printers. The higher the PPM, the faster the printer.

Several types of printers are available today, notably the dot-matrix, inkjet, laser, light-emitting diode (LED), and liquid-crystal shutter (LCS). The different printer types are also available with color-printing capability.

Color printers are more expensive than black-and-white printers. You have several alternatives when it comes to choosing a color printer:

- Color dot-matrix printers use colored ribbons to print on plain paper. A color 24-pin dot-matrix printer is your best bet for printing inexpensive, lower-quality color pages.

- Color inkjet and bubblejet printers are available for reasonably high-quality color printing on plain paper. These pages look better than color dot-matrix pages (and cost more, too).

- For laser printers, you can buy color toner cartridges, but unless you have a printer that can hold two toner cartridges at a time, you will still be printing only one color. Alternatively, you could print one color, then switch cartridges, feed the page through again, and print the second color on the same page. This process can be frustrating, as paper jams occur occasionally, forcing you to begin again.

- A color thermal-transfer printer uses heat instead of impact like the other printers mentioned above. It uses a special ribbon from which the colors melt onto the page. These are more expensive and often require special paper as well.

- The most expensive color printer is a dye sublimation printer. These are very high-quality printers, usually purchased by professional graphics artists.

Color printers are becoming more popular among general computer users. However, for many medical applications, except perhaps certain continuing medical education or patient education programs, black-and-white copies of your printed material should be adequate.

Computing Peripherals

In addition to the basic pieces of hardware discussed above, a number of computer peripherals—or extras—can also be used with your computer. Peripherals include CD-ROM drives, scanners, modems, surge protectors, and back-up devices.

CD-ROM DRIVE. A CD-ROM drive allows your computer to read a compact disc (CD) containing software or files. As has been noted, ROM stands for read-only memory because the user cannot write to the CD. A CD-ROM can hold up to approximately 600 Mb of data. Hundreds of CDs are available, ranging from the Physicians' Desk Reference and full-text medical journals to complex games and encyclopedias. (See Chapter 9 for a detailed discussion of CD-ROM technology and how it can be useful in your practice.)

SCANNER. This device records images from a printed page or from photographic film and converts them into a digital form that a computer can use and display. Scanners can be used to record images of hospital discharge summaries, electrocardiograms, or other material generated outside of your office into an electronic medical record (*see* Chapter 2).

MODEM. A modem is a device that allows a computer to send or receive data over telephone lines (*see* Chapter 8). The modem can exist as a board inside your computer or as an external device connected by a cable to your computer. A fax/modem can transmit and receive faxes as well as send or receive data. Buying a fax/modem, however, may not answer all of your facsimile needs. For example, you can send a fax only if it exists as a file in your computer—you cannot take a piece of paper and feed it into your computer to fax it somewhere (unless you have a scanner). On the other hand, a fax/modem is convenient for receiving faxes, which can be printed using your computer's printer to produce a "plain paper" fax.

SURGE PROTECTOR. A surge protector is an electrical device that goes between the wall outlet and the plug from your computer. It diffuses any surges (extra bursts of power that come through the power lines) before they can harm your computer. Most computers have a built-in surge protector, but they are not very powerful. You should add a more powerful unit to better protect your machine. The critical feature of a surge protector's ability to protect your computer from power surges is the "clamping rate," which is a measure of how quickly the device begins to suppress the power burst. The clamping rate is measured in picoseconds, and the smaller the number, the better. Your surge protector should have a clamping rate of 5 picoseconds at most; less than 1 picosecond is ideal. A good warranty is also an important feature; you should look for at least a 5-year minimum, but a lifetime warranty is most desirable.

Like the computer, a modem can be damaged by power surges, in this case surges that run through the telephone line. You should consider buying a similar device to protect your modem from these surges. Two-in-one surge protectors, with outlets for your electrical cords and jacks for your telephone wires, are available.

Backing Up Your Data

Backing up data ensures the security of your documents. Various factors can destroy data: computer viruses, hardware or software failure, environmental hazards, and mistakes. No matter how careful you are, eventually you will lose something, perhaps one small (but important) file or the contents of an entire hard disk. Making sure that you have a current set of back-up copies of important data on your hard disk helps prevent this loss from being a catastrophe.

BACK-UP MEDIA AND DEVICES. You can back up your data onto various media products, ranging from floppy disks to digital tape. You should assess the storage capacity needed, along with convenience and price, of both the storage medium and the device that copies your data onto the storage medium. Following is a list of some of the available back-up media and their storage capacities:

Back-up Medium	Storage Capacity
High-density floppy diskettes	1.4 Mb
Flopticals	21 Mb
Syquest removable cartridges	44, 88, 105, or 210 Mb

Back-up Medium	Storage Capacity
Bernoulli removable cartridges	90 and 150 Mb
3.5-inch optical disk	128 and 256 Mb
5.25-inch optical disk	650 Mb, and 1 and 1.3 Gb
Removable hard disk	Up to 1.6 Gb
Recordable CD	650 Mb
Digital tape	2 to 9 Gb

Tasks such as literature and other database searching generally do not require extensive data back-up; you may just want to periodically back up items of interest that you have retrieved and saved from your searches. If, on the other hand, you are computerizing your practice management or medical record functions, then regular back-ups to high-capacity storage media are critical.

BACK-UP PROCEDURES. In addition to some type of back-up medium, a back-up utility program is something you may want to purchase. Back-up utility software makes backing up the contents of your hard disk easier because it compresses your files (which saves space on your back-up medium); the utility software also keeps track electronically of which files are backed up and where they are on the back-up medium (tasks that may become unwieldy when done manually).

There are two types of back-up procedure: *global* and *incremental*. A global back-up is a mirror image of everything on your hard drive. An incremental back-up copies only those items that have changed since the previous global back-up. You perform a global back-up much less frequently than an incremental back-up. Back-up utilities can automate or simplify both of these procedures.

When choosing a back-up program, make certain that it works with the medium you have chosen (for example, not all back-up programs work with tape drives). Actually seeing the program work would be helpful because some are easier to use than others. Also, look at the speed at which the program backs up data. Three popular backup programs are Fastback Plus, Norton Utilities, and Retrospect.

Purchasing a Computer

You can buy computer hardware and software from various sources. It usually pays to shop around. Do not automatically ignore a smaller company with slightly higher prices—sometimes you will get a lot of attention and very good service for just a fraction more money. The kind of step-by-step approach given in Chapter 1 for implementing practice management software has much to offer in relation to the purchase of general computer hardware, too. Table 11-1 lists some of the pros and cons associated with the different purchasing options.

Understanding Software

Operating-system software was described earlier in Bits, Bytes, and Other Buzzwords. Application software—the programs you choose to accomplish specific tasks—is discussed in this section.

Table 11-1. Where To Purchase a Computer

Place	Positives	Negatives
Computer stores	You can usually test the type of computer you are buying. Often there is after-sale service and training available at the store. Warranties available.	Smaller stores have smaller selections and usually slightly higher prices.
Computer superstores	Bigger selection. Lower prices. Warranties available.	Sometimes the salespeople are not very experienced. Service and training may not be available.
Mail-order	Lowest prices. Largest selection. Quick delivery. Warranties available.	You cannot test the equipment before purchasing it. Variable service availability. Small mail-order companies come and go; exercise caution.
Newspaper classified ads (for used equipment)	Resale prices can be very low— usually less than 65% of the cost of new equipment of the same caliber.	You have no way of truly evaluating the equipment before buying and using it. No warranties.

When choosing software, you must think about what you want to accomplish with your computer. The other chapters in this book should guide you to focus on the kinds of medical programs that may be helpful in your practice. For nonmedical programs, popular magazines such as *MacWorld, PC Computing, MacUser, PC Magazine,* and *Home Office Computing* offer comparative software reviews and can be a helpful source of basic information about general-purpose computer software.

Application software can be purchased from your local computer store or a computer superstore or through mail-order (Table 11-1). Quite often, the best software bargains (and some hardware bargains, too) come from mail-order catalogs such as *The Mac Zone, The PC Zone, Mac Warehouse, Micro Warehouse,* and *MacMall* (*see* Appendix, Chapter 11, for telephone numbers).

Types of Software

Besides the wide range of clinical information management programs that are described throughout this book, many types of nonmedical software are useful for personal as well as professional endeavors. Many word processing, spreadsheet, and database programs, as well as other popular types, have been designed to make everyday tasks easier and more efficient. Specific types of practical software applications available for your computer include address-book and date-book programs, financial programs, games, project management software, and much more.

Word Processing

Word processing software greatly improves the ease with which you can create, edit, store, and retrieve text documents. A simple, inexpensive program can be used to create patient-reminder letters, information sheets, consultation reports, and other such documents. Many sophisticated programs check spelling and grammar, create tables, manipulate graphics, do mail merges, make mailing envelopes, and create informational brochures and newsletters.

Microsoft Word and WordPerfect are two of the most popular word processing programs available today. Both are available for DOS, Windows, and Macintosh platforms. Both are rich with features to make word processing easy, and increasingly, these programs give the user visual design capabilities approaching those of the special-purpose desktop publishing programs.

Spreadsheet

A spreadsheet program allows you to create an electronic balance sheet and perform intricate mathematical and statistical operations quickly and easily. You can use a spreadsheet program for your bookkeeping and accounting functions and for long-term scheduling as well. More sophisticated programs can create pie charts, bar graphs, and slides.

Two of the most popular spreadsheet programs are Microsoft Excel and Lotus 1-2-3. Both are available for Windows and Macintosh platforms, and both are rich with features to make the creation and manipulation of spreadsheet data easy.

Database

Database software helps you organize and retrieve data. The key features of a database can be compared to a traditional address book. Names and addresses are stored alphabetically with each person's listing, or *record,* containing the same categories of information, or *fields:* first name, last name, address, city, state, zip code, and telephone number. Using a computer database, you can reorganize and retrieve this data by state, zip code, first name, and so on. With commercial programs, it is straightforward to create simple databases to organize your reprint file (record = article; fields = article title, author, publication name, and so on) or track patient information (record = one patient's information; fields = patient name, patient ID, problem list, medications, and so on). A symptom, illness, medication, or anything you choose might also be designated as a field, and your records can be sorted accordingly.

Special bibliographic database management programs for filing your literature citations are described in Chapter 3 and electronic medical record programs are discussed in Chapter 2. Microsoft Access and Claris FileMaker Pro are two popular general-purpose database programs available for both Windows and Macintosh platforms.

Presentation

Presentation software lets you quickly and easily create slides, overheads, or on-screen presentations. With many of these programs, you can also create charts and utilize color beautifully; and they come with templates, so you do not have to be an artist to create an artistic presentation. Such software is a powerful aid for creating lecture, conference, and classroom presentations.

Microsoft PowerPoint and Aldus Persuasion are two popular presentation programs. Both are available for Windows and Macintosh platforms, and both are rich with features to make creating a dynamic presentation easy.

Communications

A large and growing body of information, education, and communication opportunities is accessible via telecommunications technology. Chapter 8 discusses many of these resources and how to access them. Using a modem, a telephone line, and communications software, you can discuss clinical and other matters with physicians worldwide; you can search for information on computers around the world; and you can use the value-added services of numerous online vendors. You can also send and receive faxes or data files using your computer.

When purchasing modems, remember that faster (14 400 bps or higher) is better. When you buy a modem, telecommunications software is usually also supplied. Some online services provide their own software for connecting to their system. Popular generic communications software includes CrossTalk for the PC and White Knight for the Mac.

Desktop Publishing and Illustration

If you want to publish a newsletter or create posters, flyers, brochures, or other patient education materials, you can use desktop publishing software, which has an advantage over word processing software because of its flexibility in merging and manipulating text and graphics. PageMaker and QuarkXPress, each available for both the Mac and PC, are two of the best desktop publishing programs. Another type of program, *illustration* software, gives even non-artists a chance to create dynamic graphics. These graphics can then be printed or incorporated in desktop publishing or word processing files.

Virus Protection

In computer parlance, a virus is software that is written expressly to damage computer systems. Although it may be benign, a virus can destroy the data stored on your computer, keep you from accessing your data files, or otherwise corrupt your system. Your computer can "catch" a virus from an infected floppy disk, online via a modem, or through a network. In general, you must run a program to activate a virus. Thus, you cannot catch any of the known viruses simply by reading downloaded e-mail.

For example, a physician receives a disk in the mail from a colleague. The disk contains a utility program for calculating various physiologic parameters and—often unbeknownst to the sender—a virus. The physician inserts the disk into his computer and copies the utility (and unwittingly the virus) onto his hard disk, which is networked to 20 other computers in the office. When the utility is run, the virus is activated. Since viruses usually do not start destroying things immediately, she or he may not realize that anything is wrong. However, within a few days the virus has spread via the network throughout all the computers in the building.

Obviously, viruses have the potential to cause catastrophic damage, but luckily, virus protection programs are available. Most virus protection programs locate and destroy known viruses. A popular virus protection program for the Macintosh is Symantec Antivirus for the Mac (SAM). Version 6.x of MS-DOS has a built-in virus protection program. Central Point's Anti-Virus for Windows is an alternative for use with Windows. Many large online services regularly screen their systems for viruses. In fact, Disinfectant is an excellent anti-virus program which can be downloaded from the Internet free of charge.

Utility Programs

A utility is a small program used to enhance your computer work environment. For example, in both Macintosh and Windows platforms, screen-saver utilities are available. A screen saver helps to prevent an image on your monitor from "burning" into the screen permanently, which could happen as a result of leaving an image on-screen for an extended period of time. Windows comes with a built-in screen saver. A popular and amusing alternative for both Windows and Macintosh is AfterDark. AfterDark comes with many different modules from which to choose—an aquarium, flying toasters, barking dogs, mewing kittens, bouncing balls, and so forth. These moving images help protect the screen. Additionally, many screen-saver utilities also incorporate computer security into their program, for example, password-protecting your computer whenever the screen saver starts.

Norton Utilities is a popular collection of small programs, all of which help you manage your computer. The set includes utilities for protecting and recovering data, diagnosing and repairing disk problems, and performing back-ups. Utilities enabling you to "unerase" files that were accidentally erased can come in handy and are available in Norton

Utilities and others for both the PC and Mac. Also included in Norton Utilities are tools that help optimize a system's speed and efficiency.

Copyright Issues

You should note that in most cases it is illegal to "borrow" or copy someone else's commercial software. Making illegal copies of commercial software, or "software piracy," may seem harmless, but it is unlawful and can carry stiff penalties. Commercial software usually comes in a sealed envelope that details the licensing agreement under which you may use the software.

It makes a lot of sense to legally purchase your software—you get the documentation that comes with the software, are notified when the software is updated, and receive information and "fixes" if a problem is discovered. In many cases, if you are a "registered user," you can also obtain telephone support for the program.

Some types of software—*shareware, freeware,* and *public-domain* software—can be borrowed or shared. Shareware is software that you can try before you decide to buy it. Available through online services, bulletin boards, and user groups, shareware usually costs less than $20. Freeware is software made available to the public for free by the author. The author retains the copyright to the program, so it cannot be modified in any way. Freeware is available through online services, bulletin boards, and user groups. Public-domain software is free to the public. The author gives up all rights to the program, which means anyone can modify it. Public-domain software is also available through online services, bulletin boards, and user groups.

Understanding File Storage

Files

A software application usually contains several related files. For example, word processing programs usually come with several files: the program itself, a dictionary, a thesaurus, a glossary, sample files, and preference files.

The documents you create with your computer are also stored in files. Thus, a file might contain a reminder letter, the results of a literature search, an appointment book, a consultation report received via e-mail, or a case analysis from a diagnostic decision support program. For documents that you create or load onto your hard drive, floppy diskette, or other storage location, you can determine how those files are organized.

Directories and Subdirectories

In the "paper" world, we store documents in filing cabinets. In those filing cabinets are hanging file folders and, inside them, manila folders that help organize individual papers so that they may be located again when necessary. In the electronic world, information is organized in essentially the same way.

On a PC, files are stored in directories and subdirectories. Think of directories as hanging file folders, and think of subdirectories as manila folders that are subcategories stored within a hanging file folder. Any directory or subdirectory can hold other

directories or files, or both. Thus, your entire hard drive (or floppy diskette) would be analogous to the entire file drawer. Keep track of computer files in a manner that makes sense to you. For example, you might create three main directories: one each for clinical computing resources, general computing resources, and word processing documents. You could then further organize files and program files within those directories by creating subdirectories for each program or document type. Keep in mind that the PC requires that certain operating system files and directories be available for the system to operate, so be careful not to relocate these as you personalize your directory structure.

On a Macintosh, files are organized and stored in the same way, except that the language is different. Macintosh users use *folders* to store their files. Macintosh folders can hold other folders that can hold other folders, and so on. Any folder can hold other folders or files, or both. Special files and folders needed by the operating system must also be kept in the Mac "filing cabinet."

What To Purchase: The Bottom Line

A natural reaction to the material in this chapter is indecision: There is still the question of "what should I buy?" Unfortunately, to fully answer this is difficult for two reasons. First, vastly different hardware requirements are needed to run different software programs, including those mentioned in this book. Second, software requires more space and power as it becomes increasingly sophisticated, and at the same time, hardware prices fall while power increases. Thus, any configurations recommended in this book will likely be obsolete by the time these pages are read. Leafing through a current mail-order catalog or a PC or Macintosh magazine (*see* Appendix, Chapter 11) is perhaps the best way to get a handle on current system configurations and their prices.

With these considerations in mind, several generalizations based on the state of the art in hardware and software may provide useful guideposts. In general, the types of medical applications discussed in this book (other than medical records and practice management systems) do not require the fastest, state-of-the-art devices to provide acceptable performance. In most cases, middle-of-the-road offerings will be adequate for your needs. Multimedia systems, on the other hand, require a faster, higher-end computer to optimize the processing of video material.

Here is what you need to know before you start shopping for your computer system.

PROCESSOR. The types of new PCs and Macs available today generally come with CPU chips that have adequate processing speed to provide acceptable performance on most of the medical applications described in this book.

MEMORY. The more working memory your computer has, the easier it will be to run multiple applications simultaneously on your system. For example, both Macintoshes and PCs are available with 4 Mb of RAM; but if your computer has 8 Mb, the same machines will enable you to work with several "open" applications more quickly and efficiently.

STORAGE CAPACITY. The more hard-disk storage capacity your computer has, the greater the number of programs and documents you will be able to keep on your system. Many general-purpose software products (for example, spreadsheets and word processors) require 15 to 30 or more Mb of storage space for all their program files. Some medical applications, especially those involving large databases or knowledge bases, can also approach this size. Several large applications would rapidly fill a 120-Mb hard disk, not even considering any data files that you create and may want to save. Thus, estimates of how much storage space you need should consider both the size of the applications you anticipate using and the size of the files you expect to generate for some time.

MONITOR. With a desktop computer, you should buy a color monitor. The Super VGA-type will give you the most appealing image. Fourteen inches is a popular size, but you might want to invest in a larger monitor if you will be spending prolonged periods looking at the screen or if you will be using multimedia applications frequently.

KEYBOARD. This generally comes with your computer system; you should make sure it has a comfortable touch for you.

MOUSE. This also generally comes with the system. Any basic model will get you started.

PRINTER. The black-and-white inkjet and laser printers are currently popular and adequate for most of the applications discussed in this book.

MODEM. With modems, faster is better; 14 400 bits per second is currently the slowest speed worth considering. But as speeds increase and prices fall, this lower limit is rapidly increasing.

CD-ROM DRIVE. These devices are also getting faster and better, and currently a "double-speed" device provides adequate performance and is probably the slowest worth considering. (Since software applications and databases are becoming so large, many are coming out on CD-ROM—a trend that may mitigate to some degree the need for large hard-disk capacity to store multiple programs.)

Armed with the material in this chapter and this summary of bottom-line considerations, you are ready to begin building your system. However, be assured that within 6 months or so new devices will be available that are better, faster, and cheaper. The good news is that powerful hardware, adequate to meet all the needs that most clinicians are likely to encounter at present, is readily available within financial reach. We hope that the material presented throughout this book has convinced you that now is the time to take the plunge!

Glossary

Note: *Italicized* terms also appear as main entries in the glossary.

active matrix display
A type of high-quality, full-color *LCD* (liquid-crystal display) screen used in some *notebook computers*; high resolution is achieved because a separate transistor is used to control each of the screen's *pixels*.

adapter
An interface card for personal computers; see *board*.

Apple
The company that manufactures Macintosh computers. These computers are sometimes called Apples.

application software
A program or a set of instructions that allows the computer to perform a particular function. There are general-purpose applications such as *word processing, spreadsheet,* and *database* programs and special-purpose applications, including the medically oriented software discussed in this book.

ASCII
Pronounced "as-key"; a coding system for nonformatted data that was designed to facilitate information exchange between different types of computer equipment and different computer programs; stands for American Standard Code for Information Interchange.

back up
To make a copy of a program or other data on a separate storage medium to ensure against loss of or damage to the original. Information on a *hard disk* is often backed up on a *floppy disk.*

baud
A unit of electrical oscillation in a communications signal that is used to measure speed of data transmission. Baud rate, the number of oscillations per second in a communications channel, is not necessarily equivalent to bits per second (*bps*).

bit
The smallest informational unit processed by a computer; in the computer's language, which consists of two characters, this unit of information is represented by either a zero (0) or a one (1). Eight bits grouped together compose a *byte*. Bit is a contracted form of the term "binary digit."

board
A printed circuit board containing chips and other components inserted as a removable unit in a computer or peripheral device to enable the performance of certain kinds of functioning (for example, graphics or communications); also referred to as an *adapter* or an *interface* card.

bookmark
In word processing and other applications, a function used to mark a location in a document to expedite subsequent return to that location.

Boolean search
A method of information searching in which the search terms are combined by the Boolean operators "and," "or," and "not" for, respectively, limiting, expanding, and excluding material to be retrieved by the search.

bps
Abbreviation for bits per second; a measurement of data transmission speed. In *telecommunications,* the speed at which a *modem* or *network* can transmit data over telephone lines or other channels; bps is not always equal to *baud* rate.

browsing
Searching either purposefully or aimlessly through directories, file contents, *database* information, or any other type of computer document or listing.

bug
An error in a software program or computer system that causes a malfunction.

bus
A set of parallel wires connecting computer components and devices and serving as a common distribution pathway for transmitting data.

byte
A group of eight *bits* representing a single informational unit; roughly the equivalent of a single character, for example, a letter or a numeral. Bytes are grouped together as *kilobytes* (Kb), *megabytes* (Mb), and *gigabytes* (Gb).

card
See *board.*

CD
Abbreviation for compact disc; a high-capacity storage medium using optical technology on a 4.75-inch plastic platter that stores up to 72 minutes of music or over 600 megabytes of digital information.

CD-ROM
Abbreviation for compact disc–read-only memory; a high-capacity information storage device that cannot be modified by the user. This type of CD can store the equivalent of 300 000 double-spaced, typed pages and is used on a *CD-ROM drive* to display *multimedia* material, reference books, and other information.

CD-ROM drive
An internal mechanism or *peripheral device* that enables a computer to read a compact disc holding software or files.

cell
In a *spreadsheet* grid or a table, a single box as delineated by the intersection of a column with a row.

central processing unit
Abbreviated CPU; the electronic *chip,* or micro-processor, that is the "brain" of the computer. The entire box housing the CPU chip, *hard disk, floppy-disk drive,* and other components is also referred to as the CPU.

CGA
Abbreviation for color graphics adapter; an all-but-outmoded type of computer monitor.

chip
An electronic component consisting of thousands of transistors forming an integrated circuit capable of storing and processing large amounts of information; a building block of the computer's circuitry and computational functioning.

client
In a *network,* the individual user or workstation requesting the information or resources held by the *host computer* or *server.*

client-server architecture
In a *network,* the relationship between the *local* user(s), or *client(s),* and the *host computer* (or *server*) in which the host provides the user with a range of system functionality, including software and databases.

clone
Used in reference to a *PC* made by a company other than IBM; its components and programs are all *IBM-compatible.* Also refers to recently introduced computers made by vendors other than Apple and capable of running Macintosh software.

command-line interface
The on-screen presentation of a *cursor* prompt for the user to enter an instruction, or command, by typing at the keyboard. (Compare with *graphical user interface.*)

compression software
A type of *utility* program designed to reduce a file's storage size requirement and hence effectively increase disk storage capacity.

controlled vocabulary
A list of specific terms that have a very specific meaning within an application and thereby facilitate information processing; controlled vocabularies can be used to enumerate allowable symptom or disease names in diagnostic decision support systems or medical records. (See also *data dictionary* and *structured text.*)

conversion software
A program designed to change information from one type of representation to another, such as from one computer platform to another (for example, from Mac to IBM) or from one word processing program to another (for example, from Word to WordPerfect).

CPU
Abbreviation for *central processing unit.*

cursor
On a computer monitor, a blinking symbol that indicates where the next on-screen character that the user types will appear.

data dictionary
A file, or group of files, that defines the variables and other elements used in a *database* management system such as an electronic medical record. (See also *controlled vocabulary*.)

database
Any searchable collection of information on any subject. A database program is a type of *application software* designed to manage information by organizing it into groups (or *records*) that are divided into categories (or *fields*) of data. The format is designed to provide maximum efficiency in sorting and accessing desired information. A collection of names, addresses, and telephone numbers in an address book is a classic example of a database.

decision support
Loosely refers to information systems, typically automated, that assist decision makers in gathering or analyzing, or both, information useful in making important decisions.

desktop publishing
The process of designing printed documents, often with special software applications called page-layout programs, on a personal computer.

disc
Nonmagnetic data storage medium using laser technology for *writing* and *reading* information. By convention, *optical discs* (laser based) are denoted by the word "disc"; magnetic *floppy* and *hard disks* are denoted by the word "disk."

disk
Magnetic medium for data storage; see *floppy disk* and *hard disk*. (Compare with *disc*.)

disk drive
A mechanical component in the computer, or an external component connected to the computer, which serves to rotate disks in order that data may be retrieved from storage or stored from working memory. Three types are *floppy-* and *hard-disk drives* and *CD-ROM drives*.

document
Any electronic or printed collection of text or other information; an electronic document is stored in a computer *file*.

DOS
Acronym for disk operating system. (See *MS-DOS*.)

download
To transfer data from a *host computer* system such as a network *server* or to a *client* computer such as a desktop or portable computer; to transfer data from a personal computer to a laser printer.

DPI

Abbreviation for dots per inch, a measure of image resolution used in reference to the quality of screen images and of printed matter.

drive

See *disk drive*.

e-mail

Short for electronic mail, a communication service in which messages are directed from one computer to another for retrieval by an addressee; used among participants on local, wide-area, and global *networks*.

EGA

Abbreviation for enhanced graphics adapter; an obsolete type of computer monitor.

expansion board

A printed circuit, or electronic card, that can be added to a computer to provide enhanced capability or additional functions such as expanded memory, enhanced graphics, and *modem* operation.

extended memory

In *IBM-compatible* computers, the amount of *random-access memory* in excess of the 1 megabyte that is factory-installed on the primary system *board* of the computer.

fax/modem

A modem which is also capable of sending and receiving faxes to and from a regular fax machine and other computers with a fax/modem.

field

In a *database,* an organizational category of data that forms part of a *record* of information on a particular subject; for example, in an address-book database, each record might contain separate fields for name, street address, city, state, zip code, and telephone number. (See also *record*.)

file

Generally, a collection of related data used as a basic unit of information storage; as with printed material, files are the storage units for *documents*. In electronic storage, a group of related files may compose a directory, subdirectory, or folder.

file server

A primary computer in a *network* that stores data files and applications for use by other computers in the network. The file server functions in a network as the *hard disk* functions in an individual computer.

firmware

Factory-installed software that is embedded in the *read-only memory* chips of a computer's integrated circuitry and used for the computer's systems operations.

floppy disk

A flexible, portable magnetic *disk* used for storing and transferring data, available in a 3.5-inch size (for both Macintosh and IBM-compatible computers) and a 5.25-inch size (for *IBM-compatibles* only). The flexible 3.5-inch disk is housed in a rigid plastic case. (See also *disc*.)

free text
Words not associated with any codes or structuring (as, for example, in unconstrained speaking or writing). (Compare with *structured text*.)

freeware
Software not protected by copyright and thus freely available for use and distribution by anyone.

FTP
Abbreviation for file transfer protocol. (See *protocol*.)

gateway
A connection enabling the transfer of information between two *networks* that are using different communications *protocols*.

Gb
Abbreviation for *gigabyte*.

gigabyte
Abbreviated Gb (or GB), the equivalent of 1024 *megabytes*, and often called a "gig."

GPIB
Abbreviation for general-purpose interface *bus;* a type of bus developed by Hewlett Packard (HP) to enable computers to exchange information with industrial automation equipment. Also designated *HPIB*.

graphical user interface
Abbreviated GUI; a user-friendly screen presentation that allows you to communicate with your computer by selecting *icons* and *menu* options using a pointing device such as a *mouse,* rather than entering and accessing information by typing memorized commands. (Compare with *command-line interface*.)

GUI
Pronounced "gooey," the abbreviation for *graphical user interface*.

hard disk
The magnetic data storage medium that is mounted and sealed inside the computer. Some portable computers have removable hard-disk units; supplemental, external hard-disk units are also available. The hard-disk unit has much greater storage capacity than a *floppy disk*.

hardware
A physical piece of computer system equipment, such as a monitor, *mouse,* keyboard, and printer.

host computer
In a *telecommunications network,* the central computer(s) to which individual users are connected from their *local* workstations; the server in *client-server architecture*. (See *local computer*.)

HPIB
Abbreviation for Hewlett Packard interface bus; see *GPIB*.

hypertext
A document display system that allows the user to retrieve information from a document in nonsequential order.

IBM-compatible
A *PC* made by a company other than IBM; other popular PC brands include AST, Compaq, Dell, Epson, NEC, Toshiba, and many, many more. An IBM-compatible personal computer is also called a *clone.*

icon
In a computer *interface,* a pictorial representation of an application, data file, or program function or feature; icons are characteristic of a *graphical user interface.*

information superhighway
The global array of computer *networks* used by millions of people to exchange ideas and data and to share information resources around the world. Currently, this superhighway is considered to be under construction, with only a few lanes open. The *Internet* is technically a precursor, but is sometimes used synonymously with information superhighway.

interface
The on-screen appearance of a computer application or program; the connection between the user and the program. (See *graphical user interface* and *command-line interface.*) With reference to *hardware,* interface also means the point of connection between communicating devices, for example, a *parallel port* and printer cables.

interface card
See *board.*

Internet
An international *network* of computer networks, a "system" of linked systems providing individual users with communication channels and access to software and information repositories worldwide. A forerunner of the *information superhighway,* but sometimes used synonymously.

Kb
Abbreviation for *kilobyte.*

keyword
In a database *record,* a significant term or a title of an information category that can be located and retrieved during a search procedure. Using keywords in a search on a *database* that contains a keyword *field* can improve the effectiveness of the search.

kilobyte
Abbreviated Kb (or KB), the equivalent of 1024 *bytes,* and often called a "K."

LAN
Abbreviation for *local area network.*

laptop computer
A full-featured personal computer that is small enough and light enough to be used comfortably on a person's lap; *notebook* and *subnotebook* computers, designed to be carried in a briefcase, are the smallest and lightest of these portable machines.

LCD
Abbreviation for liquid-crystal display; a technology using the reflection of light against liquid-crystal substances to create screen images in many small portable computers and other electronic devices.

local area network
Abbreviated LAN; a system of interconnected computer workstations within an office, department, or immediate neighborhood that is used for sharing application programs, files, and peripheral hardware devices.

local computer
In a *telecommunications network,* the computer used by the person connecting to the network; the client in *client-server architecture.* (See *host computer.*)

log off
To terminate a computer session, often on a client-server system; to sign off. Same as "log out."

log on
To begin a session on the computer, often within a client-server system; to sign on. Same as "log in."

Mac
Short for Macintosh, a type of personal computer that employs a *graphical user interface* and is made by Apple Computer, Inc. Macs use a different operating system and different application software from those used by *IBM-compatible* PCs. Although the Macintosh is a *personal computer,* the designation PC traditionally refers to the IBM-compatible machines.

macro
A user-created mini-program consisting of any fixed sequence of keystrokes that can be activated by a simple menu selection or a single keystroke combination. A macro is designed to eliminate the need for repetitive typing of frequently used text or formatting commands.

mainframe
Traditionally, a computer with a very large memory and storage capacity, capable of serving many users simultaneously. As *personal computers* and *networks* have become more common and powerful, they are serving many of the needs once met by mainframes.

math coprocessor
A *chip* that works with the *CPU* to accelerate mathematical calculations.

Mb
Abbreviation for *megabyte.*

medical informatics
A discipline concerned with principles and techniques related to the storage, retrieval, and use of biomedical information, data, and knowledge for problem solving and decision making.

megabyte
Abbreviated Mb (or MB); the equivalent of 1024 *kilobytes,* and often called a "meg."

memory
See *random-access memory* and *read-only memory*.

memory board
An *expansion board* that can be added to a computer to provide additional memory; also called a memory card.

memory chip
A semiconductor device that is attached to a *memory board* and stores information in the computer; *RAM* chips can be for temporary (working) storage needs, and *ROM* chips are for permanent data storage.

menu
An on-screen feature providing a list of programs, files, operations, or other options from which the user selects, directing the computer to perform a specific function.

MHz
Abbreviation for megahertz, a unit of electrical oscillation frequency applied to the measurement of computer processing speed; 1 MHz equals 1 million cycles per second.

modem
A *peripheral device* that enables a computer to send and receive data over telephone lines.

mouse
An input device that, when moved over a flat surface, positions an on-screen pointer, allowing the user to position a *cursor,* select *icons,* and perform other functions.

MS-DOS
Abbreviation for Microsoft Disk Operating System, the standard *operating system software* for IBM and *IBM-compatible* PCs.

multimedia
A format for presenting information that uses a variety of media, which may include full-motion video, sound, and still images in addition to text.

multitasking
Working at a computer with multiple programs available at the same time. Running multiple applications concurrently on the computer allows the user to quickly jump from one program to another without closing and opening applications.

network
A system of interconnected computers allowing one computer to exchange information with another computer or with another piece of peripheral equipment, for example, a printer. Networks may range in scope from the connection between two or more computers in one room, to a nationwide collection of computer systems, to a worldwide array of interconnected networks.

notebook computer
A small, portable, *laptop computer* weighing about 5 pounds and designed to fit in a briefcase.

OCR
Abbreviation for *optical character recognition.*

offline
Refers to a computer not connected via a telecommunications network to another computer (for example, a host computer). Also used in reference to *peripheral devices* (for example, printers) that are not in direct communication with a computer's *central processing unit.*

online
Refers to a computer's being "logged on" or connected via a *telecommunications* link to a *host computer,* another computer, or a *network.* Also used in reference to *peripheral devices* that are in direct communication with a computer's *central processing unit.*

operating system software
The master-control programs that run a computer and enable the use of *application software. DOS* is an example of operating system software for the *PC,* and System 7 is the current Macintosh operating system software.

optical character recognition
Abbreviated OCR; a technology whereby a printed page can be scanned (see *scanner*) or received by a *fax/modem* and converted into a *document* that can be manipulated in a *word processing application.*

optical disc
A data storage medium with very large capacity (over 600 megabytes); laser technology is used to *write* data to and *read* data from the *disc. CD-ROM* is one type of optical disc that is written to once, when it is manufactured, but can be read from repeatedly.

palmtop computer
A type of portable computing device that may be comfortably held in the hand.

parallel port
An interface terminal at the back of a computer for the simultaneous transmission of data from several channels to and from peripheral parallel devices (for example, a parallel printer).

parity
In *telecommunications,* the quality of being odd or even, used in reference to the *bits* in a segment of data transmission. A parity check is used to determine the integrity of, or freedom from error, in the unit of transmitted data.

passive matrix display
A type of *LCD* screen display used in some *notebook computers;* image quality is inferior to that provided by an *active matrix display.*

PC
Abbreviation for *personal computer.* Although Macintoshes are personal computers, the term PC by convention generally refers to an IBM or *IBM-compatible* personal computer.

PCMCIA card
A popular credit-card–sized device used with many portable and some desktop computers for expanded functions. These cards can serve as *memory, storage, modems, interfaces*, and other devices, depending on the unit. Card design adheres to the standard of the Personal Computer Memory Card International Association.

PDA
Abbreviation for *personal digital assistant*.

pen-compatible computers
Computers with a pen-sensitive drawing surface, enabling pen-based data input.

peripheral device
Any of a variety of hardware equipment, including printer, *modem, scanner,* external drive, *CD-ROM,* and others, that enable the computer to perform additional functions. A peripheral device is said to be *online* when it is in direct communication with a computer's *central processing unit.*

personal computer
Abbreviated PC; originally referred to a desktop computer designed to meet the relatively modest computing needs of an individual. As these computers have become more powerful and interconnected in networks, the distinction between personal computers and more capable workstations and *mainframe* computers is steadily blurring. (See also *PC.*)

personal digital assistant
Abbreviated PDA; a type of intermediate-sized portable computer that is small enough to be held in one hand while entering data with the other hand, often with a pen.

pixel
In a screen image, the smallest element that a monitor can display; each pixel is part of the mosaic of dots that compose the screen image.

platform
Generic term for a type of computer environment, computer system, or operating system. *Macintosh, IBM-compatible PCs,* and *UNIX* machines are examples of *hardware* platforms. *Operating system software* such as DOS and Windows are also referred to as platforms.

port
A socket or plug-in terminal at the back of a computer into which cables from *peripheral devices* are connected.

protocol
In computer parlance, a set of agreed-upon rules shared by communicating systems. For example, *FTP,* which stands for file transfer protocol, is an *Internet* tool that enables a user at his local machine to retrieve files from other computers on the Internet.

query language
A special language used to request and retrieve information from a *database* management system; standard query languages exist, but some database systems have their own query language.

RAM
Acronym for *random-access memory*.

random-access memory
Abbreviated RAM; the primary working memory in a computer that allows quick access to data; active applications and files are held in RAM. Generally, any information stored in RAM is erased when the computer is shut off.

read
To retrieve information from a *hard disk, floppy disk, CD-ROM disc* or other storage medium. (Compare with *write*.)

read-only memory
Abbreviated ROM; computer *memory* or *storage* that can be *read* but not *written* to by the user. ROM is created at the time of computer chip, card, or disc manufacture and is used to store the computer's essential system programming or other nonchangeable data.

record
In a *database,* the primary unit of organization. For example, in an address book database there might be a separate record for each entry (for example, company or person). (See also *field*.)

ROM
Acronym for *read-only memory*.

scanner
A *peripheral device* enabling the input of external images and text to a computer; a scanner records images from a printed page, photographic film, or other source and converts them into a digital form that a computer can manipulate and display.

screen saver
A *utility* that helps to prevent an image on the monitor from permanently "burning" into the screen by temporarily replacing the screen image with a moving image.

SCSI
Abbreviation for small computer systems interface (pronounced "scuzzy"); an *interface* for connecting *peripheral devices* to a *personal computer*.

search engine
A software component designed to retrieve information such as relevant passages from a reference text in accordance with user-provided instructions. Search engines often provide for several different kinds of searches, such as *Boolean searches* and *keyword* searches.

search strategy
User-created instructions entered into a *search engine* to identify and retrieve desired topics or references from a *database;* some searching programs allow search strategies to be saved for reuse at a later time.

serial port
An *interface* terminal at the back of a computer for the input and output of sequential data, that is, information that is received and transmitted one *bit* at a time.

server
In a *network,* the *host computer* or provider of databases, applications, and other resources to the *client* which is making requests for such data.

shareware
Software made available by the copyright holder for trial use by others, who may keep the product upon payment of a registration fee to the owner.

software
See *application software* and *operating system software.*

spreadsheet
A type of general-purpose *application software* designed to facilitate tabular work with numbers, including mathematical calculations and graphing operations.

start bit
In serial communications, a *bit* indicating the beginning of a data stream, or the start of a *byte* of data.

stop bit
In serial communications, the *bit* inserted at the end of a *byte* of data to indicate that the data stream is complete.

storage
The retention of data on a *hard disk, floppy disk, compact disc,* or other storage medium; a computer's capacity for program and data storage is not related to the amount of *memory (RAM)* it has for processing information.

structured text
Information whose content is organized by predefined data types and/or coded in a way that readily enables the user to locate, modify, and retrieve any particular component of the text. (See also *controlled vocabulary.*)

subnotebook computer
An ultralight portable computer that is smaller than a *notebook computer* but has a full-sized keyboard and is capable of running essentially the same programs used on desktop computers.

super VGA
Abbreviated SVGA; an advanced type of monitor offering color capability and image resolution superior to those of a standard *VGA* (video graphics adapter) monitor.

surge protector
A device placed between any computer component and the source of current (or other signals) feeding that component in order to protect the sensitive electronic circuits of the component from bursts of power that come through the electric lines (or other sources).

SVGA
Abbreviation for *super VGA.*

telecommunications
Broadly refers to electronic communications systems including telephones, but in the context of computer systems, it generally refers to information transmission via telephone lines or other channels between geographically distant computers.

UNIX
The proprietary name of a specialized type of *operating system software* designed for handling multiple users; thus, UNIX is sometimes the operating system of choice for developers of products such as practice management systems. Computers designed to run the UNIX operating system are sometimes called UNIX machines.

unstructured text
Text that does not contain embedded codes or that is not associated with predefined *fields;* also called *free text.*

upload
To transfer data to a *host computer* system from a local or *client* computer, for example, to a network *server* from a desktop computer.

user interface
The on-screen appearance, or the program component with which the user interacts by inputting data, selecting options, issuing commands, and viewing the results of these actions. User interfaces may be graphical (for example, as with Macintosh or Windows computers) or character based (for example, as with DOS or UNIX machines).

utility
A specialized computer program used to enhance a particular function or aspect of the computer work environment; for example, programs for doing automatic *back-ups,* diagnosing disk problems, detecting and eliminating *viruses,* and screen saving are all utilities.

VGA
Abbreviation for video graphics adapter; the current minimum standard for computer monitors, offering a much finer image than the outmoded *EGA* and *CGA* types; the abbreviation VGA may also be translated as video graphics array or virtual graphics array. (See also *super VGA.*)

virtual reality
Computer simulation using three-dimensional graphics as well as devices such as glove sensors and binocular television headsets so that the user can interact with the simulation in a life-like manner.

virus
A piece of software that has been written expressly to damage computer systems; generally transmitted by infected software that has been loaded from a *floppy disk* or *downloaded* from a *host computer.*

WAN
Abbreviation for *wide area network*.

wide area network
Abbreviated WAN; a system of interconnected computers encompassing a large geographic range, including cities, states, or countries. (See *network* and compare with *local area network*.)

Windows
Trademark of Microsoft Corporation, a PC operating environment used with Microsoft's MS-DOS operating system. A *graphical user interface* designed to facilitate *multitasking*; Windows is similar to the Macintosh *GUI* but uses different *application software*.

word processor
A type of *application software* that enables the user to enter, edit, and format text.

write
To use an input device such as a keyboard or *mouse* to transfer information from working memory to a storage medium such as a *hard* or *floppy disk;* also, to transfer data from working memory to the computer's display screen. (Compare with *read*.)

write protect
To protect against the inadvertent recording or modifying of data on a *floppy disk;* write protection is mechanically ensured by adjusting the position of a special tab on the floppy disk.

WYSIWYG
Abbreviation for what you see is what you get (pronounced "wizzywig"); an interface feature of *word processing* systems in which the on-screen appearance of the text is identical to that produced in the printed document.

Appendix: Information Resources

The information below is presented in parallel form with the Introduction and 11 chapters of the book.

Introduction:
Improving Clinical Information Management in Everyday Medical Practice (General Resources)

American College of Physicians (ACP)

As mentioned in the Introduction and Foreword, ACP has a strong commitment to supporting the appropriate use of information technology in clinical practice. Several products and services provided by the College are noted below. Additional information about these offerings can be obtained by calling the Customer Service department at the number listed below.

American College of Physicians
Independence Mall West
Sixth Street at Race
Philadelphia, PA 19106-1572
Telephone: 215-351-2600 or 800-523-1546,
     ext. 2600 (Customer Service)

Educational Programs

ACP ANNUAL SESSION: ACP's primary educational meeting, held in the spring of each year. Roughly 30 courses within the larger scientific program are devoted to the use of computers in practice. A Medical Informatics Resource Room is available during the meeting for hands-on experience with medically oriented products and for consultation with experts in the clinical use of computers. A pre-session course provides an in-depth introduction to using computers in practice.

POSTGRADUATE COURSES: Planned to begin in late 1995, regional courses will provide an in-depth introduction to the use of computers in clinical practice. Call Customer Service for information on course locations and dates.

Publications

THE ACP INFORMATION TECHNOLOGY SERIES: Initial titles are this book and *Software for Internists: Critical Evaluations from* Medical Software Reviews *and the Journal Literature*. Call Customer Service for information about these books.

ACP OBSERVER: A monthly news magazine for College members and other subscribers that regularly highlights topics related to the use of computers in practice. A supplement on computers in practice appears yearly.

Computer-based Information and Education Products

MKSAP 10 ELECTRONIC: Complete information from MKSAP 10 (Medical Knowledge Self-Assessment Program) available on CD-ROM. Includes the syllabus and annotated bibliographies as well as capability to answer multiple-choice questions and receive CME credit. Planned for release in Fall 1995.

ACP JOURNAL CLUB ON DISK: Complete text from *ACP Journal Club* available in two formats: as a stand-alone product on floppy disks or integrated with the full text of cited articles on CD-ROM.

ACP *CLINICAL PRACTICE GUIDELINES* ON DISK: Text from ACP's publication *Clinical Practice Guidelines,* available in either Windows or Macintosh versions. The disk features structured abstracts and guidelines only; full-text review articles are not included.

FULL TEXT OF *ANNALS OF INTERNAL MEDICINE*: *Annals* is available in full text (1991–1994 issues) on CD-ROM from Appleton and Lange New Media and Creative Multimedia. Both vendors participate in the ACP Product Discount Service (listed below). CDP Technologies (800-950-2035) provides *Annals* online.

ACP LIBRARY ON DISK: A collection of ACP's clinical information products, including *ACP Journal Club, Clinical Practice Guidelines*, the syllabus from MKSAP 10 and several subspecialty MKSAPs, and other publications, will be available on CD-ROM and searchable from a single graphical interface. Scheduled for release in early 1996.

GEOMEDICA: ACP is working with Reuters Health Information Services, Inc. (RHIS), to develop interactive multimedia continuing medical education (CME) titles. These CD-ROM–based offerings cover diverse topics in internal medicine and contain text, audio, and full-motion video material. These titles can be viewed using RHIS's GeoMedica workstation. Telephone: 800-850-2464.

Services

ACP ONLINE: An online bulletin board and information repository for ACP members. Used for communication and information exchange on clinical practice, medical education, computer use, health reform, and other topics.

PRODUCT DISCOUNT SERVICE: Medically oriented software and related products from outside vendors offered to ACP members at a discount. Call Customer Service for a copy of the ACP catalog, *Resources for Internists,* which lists participating vendors and provides ordering information.

NLM FLAT-FEE PROGRAM: ACP members receive GRATEFUL MED software and unlimited access to MEDLINE and other NLM databases for a flat fee of $200 per year.

Research and Development

ACP is actively engaged in research and development aimed at building on the collection of products and programs outlined above. The common theme of these efforts is to help physicians effectively use information technology to manage medical information. For additional information on these projects, contact the coordinator, Clinical Information Management department, at 215-351-2400; via CompuServe at mhs:medinfo@acp; or via Internet at medinfo@acp.mhs.compuserve.com

Other Associations and Societies

Many local, state, and national medical specialty societies offer various types of support to clinicians interested in using computers in their practice. In addition, the American Medical Informatics Association (AMIA), the premier medical informatics organization, is a national professional society for those interested in the use of computers in health care. AMIA has a journal (*JAMIA*) and a proceeding (SCAMC; *see under* Meetings), both indexed in MEDLINE.

American Medical Informatics Association (AMIA)
4915 St. Elmo Avenue, Suite 302
Bethesda, MD 20814
Telephone: 301-657-1291
E-mail: mail@amia2.amia.org

Resources for Identifying and Evaluating Products

Many hundreds of different medical software products are on the market. These resources vary widely in their functionality and quality. Furthermore, different products are geared toward different types of consumers, for example, physicians, non-physician health care providers, or institutions. As discussed in the Introduction to this book, colleagues, meetings, and medical centers are helpful for identifying and evaluating products useful in your practice. Listed below is a sampling of directories, catalogs, and sources of product reviews that also support clinicians in selecting and purchasing products. In addition, journals and magazines contain ads, articles, and reviews that can be helpful in these tasks.

Product Directories

The 1995 HCP Directory of Medical Software. Edited by Bruce H. Frisch. Includes basic product and company information covering medical software running on microcomputers or minicomputers and available to medical professionals. Healthcare Computing Publications Inc., 462 Second Street, Brooklyn, NY 11215. Telephone: 718-499-5910; fax: 718-768-3260.

MD Computing Annual Medical Hardware and Software Buyer's Guide (November-December issue). Telephone: 1-800-SPRINGER.

Interactive Healthcare Directories. Provides directories on topics such as CD-ROM, computer-aided instruction, and online services. Stewart Publishing, Inc., 6471 Merritt Court, Alexandria, VA 22312. Telephone: 703-354-8155.

Catalogs of Medical Computing Products

Alpha Media (800-832-1000)
Medical Software Products (800-444-4570)

Product Reviews

Medical Software Reviews. Edited by Sue Frisch. Monthly newsletter featuring independent, objective evaluations of medical software written by practicing clinicians. Healthcare Computing Publications Inc., 462 Second Street, Brooklyn, NY 11215. Telephone: 718-499-5910; fax: 718-768-3260.

Software for Internists: Critical Evaluations from Medical Software Reviews *and the Journal Literature.* Edited by Sue Frisch. Useful for identifying available products and learning about critical issues in their implementation. Readers should contact individual publishers and other sources for up-to-date product information. *Medical Software Reviews* (*see* page 217) is an excellent source for reviews of contemporary product versions. American College of Physicians, Independence Mall West, Sixth Street at Race, Philadelphia, PA 19106-1572. Telephone: 800-523-1546, ext. 2600.

In addition to reviews from these sources, many leading medical specialty journals such as the *Journal of the American Medical Association, Annals of Internal Medicine, Journal of Family Practice,* and others also periodically contain reviews of new medical computing products. The editors of *Medical Software Reviews* maintain a list of such reviews that they will send to you free on receipt of a written request.

Meetings

A growing number of meetings hosted by specialty societies (for example, ACP's Annual Session) and others feature courses on computers in medicine. These meetings often feature a vendor exhibit area that can be useful to those interested in learning about and beginning to evaluate specific products. A sampling of annual conferences in which computers in medicine is the major theme is given below.

AMIA's Symposium on Computer Applications in Medical Care (SCAMC)

This large (2000+ participants) annual scientific meeting of AMIA covers the entire field of medical informatics and is held in the late fall. AMIA's Spring Congress is a smaller scientific meeting, which focuses on a different topic in medical informatics each year.

MEDINFO

This conference is held every 3 years and is the scientific meeting of the International Medical Informatics Association (IMIA). IMIA also holds small (100+ participants) workshops, some in the U.S., on various subjects. IMIA does not have individual members; its members are countries' medical informatics organizations such as AMIA. IMIA can be reached at: 16 Place Longemalle, CH-1204 Geneva, Switzerland. Telephone: 41-22-3102649; fax: 41-22-7812322; e-mail: IFIP@CGEUGE51.bitnet

Annual Interactive Healthcare Conference

Various topics are covered at this conference, for example, telecommunications, CD-ROM, and computer-aided instruction (CAI); it is geared primarily toward educators in institutional settings. Sponsored by Stewart Publishing, Inc., 6471 Merritt Court, Alexandria, VA 22312. Telephone: 703-354-8155.

Computers in Healthcare Education

This meeting is co-sponsored each spring in Philadelphia, Pennsylvania, by the Thomas Jefferson University and the Health Sciences Library Consortium. It is designed for and by medical and allied health educators. Call 215-222-1532 for more information.

Journals and Magazines

Various periodicals focus on a wide range of topics related to computers in medicine, including institutional and physician-oriented applications, as well as the science of computers in health care (that is, medical informatics). A sampling of such publications is given below.

Scientific Journals

Canadian Medical Informatics, Hermal Vienneau, CP/PO Box 64, Bathurst, New Brunswick, Canada E2A 3Z1. Telephone: 506-546-4085.

Computers and Biomedical Research, Academic Press, 1250 Sixth Avenue, San Diego, CA 92101. Telephone: 619-699-6742.

Journal of American Medical Informatics Association (JAMIA). Telephone: 301-657-1291.

MD Computing, Springer-Verlag, Inc., 15 Fifth Avenue, New York, NY 10010. Telephone: 800-777-4643.

Magazines and Newsletters

Clinical Data Management (monthly newsletter), Aspen Publishers, Inc., 7201 McKinney Circle, Frederick, MD 21701. Telephone: 301-417-7500.

Computers and Medicine, Box 36, Glencoe, IL 60022. Telephone: 708-446-3100.

Healthcare Informatics, Health Data Analysis, Inc., P.O. Box 2830, Evergreen, CO 80439. Telephone: 303-674-2774.

Physicians and Computers, Moorhead Publications, Inc., 810 S. Waukegan Road, Suite 200, Lake Forest, IL 60045. Telephone: 708-615-8333.

Books and Articles

A diverse literature has been written dealing with information management in medicine and with the role of computers in supporting this information management. A sampling of books and articles on these topics is given below.

Blois MS. Clinical judgment and computers. N Engl J Med. 1980;303:192-7.

Blois MS. Information in Medicine: The Nature of Medical Descriptions. Berkeley, California: University of California Press; 1984.

Covell DG, Uman GC, Manning PR. Information needs in office practice: are they being met? Ann Intern Med. 1985;103:596-9.

Greenes RA, Shortliffe EH. Medical informatics. An emerging academic discipline and institutional priority. JAMA. 1990;263:1114-20.

Hersh W, Hickam D. Use of a multi-application computer workstation in a clinical setting. Bull Med Libr Assoc. 1994;82:382-9.

Osheroff JA, Bankowitz RA. Physicians' use of computer software in answering clinical questions. Bull Med Libr Assoc. 1993;81:11-9.

Osheroff JA, Forsythe DE, Buchanan BG. Physicians' information needs: analysis of questions posed during clinical teaching. Ann Intern Med. 1991;114:576-81.

Shortliffe EH, Perreault LE, Wiederhold G, Fagan LW, eds. Medical Informatics: Computer Applications in Health Care. New York: Addison-Wesley; 1990.

Williamson JW, German PS, Weiss R, et al. Health science information management and continuing education of physicians. A survey of U.S. primary care practitioners and their opinion leaders. Ann Intern Med. 1989;110:151-60.

Chapter 1. Practice Management

Identifying Additional Products for Practice Management

In addition to comprehensive practice management systems, various software products are available to support a range of management aspects of medical practice. These resources include programs for electronic claims submission, scheduling, regulation compliance, visit and procedure coding, fee calculations, billing, and office accounting. Some software directories and catalogs (*see under* Introduction in this Appendix) list products in categories such as these. Complete practice management systems as well as products in each of these categories are reviewed in detail in ACP's *Software for Internists*.

Catalogs for purchasing general hardware and supplies that can be used for practice management systems are listed under Chapter 11 in this Appendix.

Associations

Some state and county medical societies provide members with information useful for selecting from local vendors and practice management systems. Contact your regional society for additional information.

Publications

Hudson VJ. The HCP Directory of Medical Office Management Computer System Vendors with Satisfaction Ratings. 2d edition. New York: Healthcare Computing Publications Inc.; 1995. Telephone: 718-499-5910.

ASIM Computer Information Packet: A packet of materials designed to help practitioners select a practice management system. Available from the American Society for Internal Medicine (ASIM). Telephone: 202-835-2746, ext. 246.

Needle S. Guide to Medical Practice Software Management. Rockville, Maryland: CTS; 1995. Telephone: 800-433-8015; in Maryland: 301-468-4800.

Cushing M Jr. Checklist for Practice Management System Selection. Available from Healthcare Computing Publications Inc. Telephone: 718-499-5910.

Computerized Medical Office. A guide to selecting practice management systems. Available from Medicode. Telephone: 800-999-4600.

Chapter 2. Medical Record Systems for Office Practice

Identifying Additional Products for Electronic Medical Records

In addition to electronic medical record programs, various software products are available to facilitate the creation and management of various components of patient records. These include programs for gathering, organizing, and coding data from patients. Some directories and catalogs (*see under* Introduction in this Appendix) list products in categories such as these. In addition, ACP's *Software for Internists* contains detailed reviews of such products, including portable systems and systems that accept voice input.

Courses

Courses focusing on implementing electronic patient records are beginning to emerge within educational meetings on medical computing and as stand-alone courses. An example of a popular annual course on issues related to implementing medical record systems in hospital settings is "Clinical Computing in Patient Care: What the Clinician Needs To Know." This 2-day course is directed by faculty from the Harvard Medical School Center for Clinical Computing and is sponsored by AMIA. Telephone: 617-732-7928.

Other Information Resources

The Institute of Medicine (IOM), an advisory body to the federal government, convened a committee to identify strategies for improving the patient record. The recommendations of this committee are described in a landmark book:

Dick RS, Steen EB, eds. The Computer-based Patient Record: An Essential Technology for Healthcare. Committee on Improving the Patient Record, Division of Health Care Services, Institute of Medicine. Washington, D.C.: National Academy Press; 1991.

The cornerstone recommendation in this report is that "1. Healthcare professionals and organizations should adopt the computer-based patient record (CPR) as the standard for medical and all other records related to patient care." The second recommendation is "2. To accomplish Recommendation No. 1, the public and private sectors should join in establishing a Computer-based Patient Record Institute to promote and facilitate development, implementation, and dissemination of the CPR." In response to the IOM report, such an organization has been formed:

Computer-Based Patient Record Institute (CPRI)
1000 East Woodfield Road, Suite 102
Schaumburg, IL 60173
Telephone: 708-706-6746; fax: 708-706-6747

Although the primary focus of CPRI work has not specifically been on medical record systems for office practice, this organization is a useful resource for information on broader issues related to the development of computer-based patient records.

A companion volume to the IOM book on computer-based patient records contains the reports considered by the IOM committee in making their recommendations:

Ball MJ, Collen MF, eds. Aspects of the Computer-based Patient Record. Computers in Health Care Series. New York: Springer-Verlag; 1992.

The Medical Records Institute is a for-profit organization that has also focused on the development and dissemination of computer-based patient records. Their activities include an annual conference, "Toward an Electronic Patient Record," and a monthly newsletter with the same title.

Medical Records Institute
567 Walnut Street/P.O. Box 289
Newton, MA 02160
Telephone: 617-964-3923

Articles

Many articles concerning the computerization of parts or all of patient records have been published in the medical literature. A small sampling is given below.

Barnett GO, Jenders FA, Chueh HC. The computer-based clinical record—where do we stand? Ann Intern Med. 1993;119:1046-8.

McDonald CJ, Tierney WM. Computer-stored medical records: their future role in medical practice. JAMA. 1988;5:34-7.

Shortliffe EH, Tang PC, Detmer DE. Patient records and computers. Ann Intern Med. 1991;115:979-81.

Tierney WM, Miller ME, McDonald CJ. The effect on test ordering of informing physicians of the charges for outpatient diagnostic tests. N Engl J Med. 1990; 322:1499-504.

Tierney WM, Miller ME, Overhage M, McDonald CJ. Physician inpatient order writing on microcomputer workstations. JAMA. 1993;269:379-84.

Weed LL. Medical records that guide and teach. N Engl J Med. 1968;278:593-600.

Computer-based patient records can provide a platform for implementing systems for reminding clinicians about potentially beneficial but easily overlooked interventions. A growing literature documents the value of such reminder systems. Examples include:

Barnett GO. The application of computer-based medical record systems in ambulatory practice. N Engl J Med. 1984;310:1643-50.

McDonald CJ. Protocol-based computer reminders: the quality of care and the non-perfectibility of man. N Engl J Med. 1976;295:1351-5.

Chapter 3.
Medical Literature Management

Identifying Additional Products for Medical Literature Management

Various programs other than those mentioned in Chapter 3 can be useful for accessing, synthesizing, and filing medical literature. For example, the BiblioMed series of products (available from HealthCare Information Services, Inc.; 800-468-1128) offers literature citations in different areas, including gastroenterology, cardiology, urology, general medical reference, and others. QuickScan Reviews (available from Educational Reviews, Inc.; 800-633-4743) is one example of a literature synopsis program available on disk. Some medical software directories and catalogs (*see under* Introduction in this Appendix) list software in each of the product categories covered in Chapter 3. In addition, several popular literature searching and filing programs are reviewed in ACP's *Software for Internists*.

The National Library of Medicine (NLM)

The NLM has long been an international resource for biomedical literature. Besides their well-known activities in gathering, indexing, and disseminating medical literature, the NLM supports various intramural and extramural research and development projects. The common theme of all these activities is improving the management, dissemination, and use of biomedical knowledge.

National Library of Medicine
Public Information Office
8600 Rockville Pike
Bethesda, MD 20894
Telephone: 800-272-4787

A recent article highlights the role in patient care of searching NLM's MEDLINE database:

Lindberg DAB, Siegel ER, Rapp BA, Wallingford KT, Wilson SR. Use of MEDLINE by physicians for clinical problem solving. JAMA. 1993;269: 3124-9.

Chapter 4.
Diagnostic Decision Support

Identifying Additional Products for Diagnostic Decision Support

Besides the general medical diagnostic systems discussed in Chapter 4, various available programs support diagnosis in specific topic areas such as psychiatry, dermatology, obesity etiology, sleep disor-

ders, and laboratory abnormalities. Some medical software directories and catalogs (*see under* Introduction in this Appendix) contain a separate section for diagnostic support systems. Reviews of several general and topical diagnostic programs can be found in ACP's *Software for Internists*.

Besides stand-alone diagnostic systems, products that integrate diagnostic support with other clinical information management functionality are beginning to appear in greater number. For example, Medical Consult '95 is a new software program available from Blackwell Science, Inc. (800-215-1000), that succinctly provides information and recommendations from experts on diagnosing and treating clinical problems for which consultation is frequently requested. Similarly, Problem Knowledge Couplers (PKC Corporation; 800-752-5351) also provide integrated diagnostic and therapeutic support (*see under* Chapter 5 in this Appendix).

Increasingly, diagnostic resources such as Medical Consult '95, QMR (*see* Chapter 4), and others are available for small, portable computers. (*See under* Chapter 10 in this Appendix for information on identifying software products for portable computers.)

Articles

Much has been published in the medical literature on the promise and challenges of diagnostic decision support systems. A sampling of such articles, focusing on the systems discussed in Chapter 4, is presented below.

Bankowitz RA, McNeil MA, Challinor SM, et al. A computer-assisted medical diagnostic consultation service: implementation and prospective evaluation of a prototype. Ann Intern Med. 1989;110:824-32.

Barnett GO, Cimino JJ, Hupp JA, Hoffer EP. DXplain: an evolving diagnostic decision-support system. JAMA. 1987;258:67-74.

Bergeron B. Iliad: a diagnostic consultant and patient simulator. MD Computing. 1991;8:46-53.

Berner ES, Webster GD, Shugerman AA, et al. Performance of four computer-based diagnostic systems. N Engl J Med. 1994;330:1792-6.

Carter J. Diagnostic support: DXplain, Iliad, QMR (a comparative review). Medical Software Reviews. 1994;3:1-4. (Reprint available free on receipt of a written request to Healthcare Computing Publications Inc. *See under* Introduction, Product Reviews, in this Appendix for address.)

Johnston ME, Langton KB, Haynes RB, Mathieu A. Effects of computer-based clinical decision support systems on clinician performance and patient outcome. A critical appraisal of research. Ann Intern Med. 1994;120:135-42.

Kassirer JP. A report card on computer-assisted diagnosis—the grade: C [Editorial]. N Engl J Med. 1994; 330:1824-5.

Miller RA, Masarie F. The demise of the "Greek Oracle" model for medical diagnostic systems. Meth Inform Med. 1990;29:1-2.

Waxman HS, Worley WE. Computer-assisted adult medical diagnosis: subject review and evaluation of a new microcomputer-based system. Medicine. 1990; 69:125-36.

Chapter 5.
Therapeutic Decision Support

Identifying Additional Products for Therapeutic Decision Support

As covered in this book, the topic of therapeutic decision support (TDS) refers to a loose collection of more specific technologies for tasks such as obtaining drug information, prescription writing and tracking, drug interaction detection, and others. In part, because TDS comprises many discrete topics, there is a paucity of supplemental resources focusing broadly on electronic information products for the entire area. However, some medical software directories and catalogs (*see under* Introduction in this Appendix) list products in these component areas.

Several individual products for therapeutic decision support are mentioned in Chapter 5. Many of these programs, as well as others including various diet therapy products, are reviewed in ACP's *Software for Internists*.

Innovative applications that integrate therapeutic support with other clinical information management functions are emerging. One thoughtful and relatively unique approach is embodied in Problem Knowledge Couplers available from PKC Corporation (800-752-5351). Developed by Lawrence Weed and colleagues, these programs build on Dr. Weed's pioneering work developing the S-O-A-P (subjective-objective-assessment-plan) format for patient records. Problem Knowledge Couplers are Microsoft Windows-based, point-of-care clinical decision support tools for identifying patient problems, eliciting and recording patient findings, and refining diagnostic and management strategies. Medical Consult '95 is an example of another new application that merges diagnostic and therapeutic support (*see under* Chapter 4 in this Appendix).

As with diagnostic decision support programs, therapeutic support programs are increasingly available for small portable computing devices. (*See under* Chapter 10 in this Appendix for information on identifying software for these devices.)

Scientific evaluations of computer-based clinical decision support systems have matured to the point where a provocative review of controlled trials has recently been published:

> Johnston ME, Langton KB, Haynes RB, Mathieu A. Effects of computer-based clinical decision support systems on clinician performance and patient outcome: a critical appraisal of research. Ann Intern Med. 1994;120:135-42.

Chapter 6. Patient Education

Identifying Additional Products for Patient Education

Various programs exist, other than those mentioned in Chapter 6, for educating patients about diagnoses and therapies, discharge instructions, informed consent issues, and the like. Some products work as modules of medical record or practice management systems; some are designed for use by patients in their homes; and others are stand-alone applications used in the physician's office. Medical software catalogs and directories (*see under* Introduction in this Appendix) can be a good source for identifying individual products of each type. The Informed Patient Decisions Group (*see under* Other Information Resources) publishes a directory of software for patient education. Various patient education programs are also evaluated in ACP's *Software for Internists*.

Other Information Resources

Increasing attention is being focused on using computer technology to educate patients, and various resources are available to support such education.

The Health Commons Institute is a non-profit organization, which focuses on promoting the use of information technology to improve patient education within the doctor-patient relationship. They offer a newsletter, reference materials, and conferences on this topic.

Health Commons Institute
50 Monument Square, Suite 500
Portland, ME 04101
Telephone: 207-874-6552

The Informed Patient Decisions Group is a university-based team involved in evaluating and promoting technologies which enhance patient education. They publish a directory of patient education software.

Informed Patient Decisions Group
Oregon Health Sciences University MC BICC-504
3181 S.W. Sam Jackson Park Road
Portland, OR 97201-3098
Telephone: 503-494-4808

The National Council on Patient Information and Education (NCPIE) is a non-profit coalition of more than 375 health care organizations committed to improving communication between patients and health care professionals about prescription medicines. Their directory of available products includes a variety of software, including CD-ROM products.

National Council on Patient Information and
    Education (NCPIE)
666 Eleventh Street NW, Suite 810
Washington, DC 20001
Telephone: 202-347-6711

The Institute for International Research (IRI) sponsored a conference in December 1994 titled "Multimedia Patient Education: Enabling Technologies for Clinical and Managed Care Practices." Information on transcripts and audio tapes of the conference can be obtained from IRI by telephone at 800-345-8016.

Patient Education Resources Accessible Online

A growing collection of information useful for educating patients is available from online sources such as bulletin boards, value-added services such as America Online, and on the Internet. A small sample of addresses for such resources on the Internet is listed below. (*See under* Chapter 8 in this Appendix for an explanation of URL, or universal resource locator.)

Medical College of Wisconsin's International
    Travelers Clinic
URL: http://www.intmed.mcw.edu/travel.html

New York State Education and Research Network
    Breast Cancer Information Clearing House
URL: http://nysernet.org/breast/Default.html

National Cancer Institute's patient information
    sheets
URL: http://biomed.nus.sg:80/Cancer/PhyPat.html

Articles

The articles below illustrate early work on patient-computer interaction as well as recent literature overviews on using computers to help educate patients.

Kahn G. Computer-generated patient handouts. MD Computing. 1993;10;157-64.

Kahn G. Computer-based patient education: a progress report. MD Computing. 1993;10;93-9.

Slack WV, Hicks PG, Reed CE, Van Cura LJ. A computer-based medical history system. N Engl J Med. 1966;274:194-8.

Chapter 7. Personal Continuing Medical Education

Identifying Additional Products and Resources for CME

Practitioners interested in CME applications for personal use will find general medical software catalogs and directories (*see under* Introduction in this Appendix) and medical CD-ROM catalogs (*see under* Chapter 9 in this Appendix) useful for identifying available products. Various programs for both CME and undergraduate and graduate medical education are discussed in ACP's *Software for Internists*.

A promising trend in CME is the emergence of medical information management programs that offer

AMA Category 1 credit. UpToDate in Nephrology and Hypertension is one example discussed in Chapter 7; another example is QuickScan Reviews, noted under Chapter 3 in this Appendix.

Other resources for identifying education software, geared primarily to the undergraduate and graduate levels, include the following:

Health Sciences Libraries Consortium: Computer Based Learning Software for Healthcare Education (a software catalog), 3600 Market Street, Philadelphia, PA 19104. Telephone: 215-222-1532.

Interactive Healthcare Directory: Computer Assisted Instruction, Stewart Publishing. Telephone: 703-354-8155.

Software for Health Sciences Education: A Resource Catalog, available from the Learning Resource Center, Office of Medical Education, University of Michigan Medical School, Ann Arbor, MI 48109-0726.

Maintenance of Competence Program (MOCOMP)

MOCOMP is an innovative Canadian CME initiative that emphasizes continuing professional development through identifying, recording, and addressing the information needs that arise during patient care (*see* Chapter 7).

MOCOMP
The Royal College of Physicians and Surgeons
  of Canada
774 Echo Drive
Ottawa, Canada K1S 5N8
Telephone: 613-730-6243 or 800-461-9598;
  fax: 613-730-0500

Chapter 8. Telecommunications

Background: Internet Addresses

This section provides some additional background information to help those new to computer communications access the Internet resources discussed in Chapter 8 and in this Appendix.

Structure of an Internet E-mail Address

Most personal Internet e-mail addresses contain two parts connected by an "@" and strung together without any spaces. These parts consist of the person's name or user ID and the address of their host computer system.

The typical Internet e-mail address has the form: userID@hostname.domain

An example is: Klee0002@student.tc.umn.edu

The host computer on which you have an account has a name known as the "hostname." Other computers on the Internet identify your host computer by this name. The hostname is important whenever you wish to communicate with someone who is connected to another host. In the example above, the hostname is "student.tc.umn". A code indicating the "domain" or classification of the host computer makes up the last portion of the e-mail address. At one time, only a few domains existed: .EDU (educational institutions); .COM (commercial organizations); .GOV (government organizations); .MIL (military); .NET (network organizations); and .ORG (non-profit organizations), to name a few. Now there are many more. As of January 1995, there were 242 domain names for countries around the world, from .AD (Andorra) to .US (United States) to .ZW (Zimbabwe).

Accounts on host systems that are not part of the Internet proper (for example, CompuServe, Prodigy, and America Online) generally have their own format for e-mail addresses. However, most of these systems have "gateways" to the Internet that enable the bi-directional exchange of e-mail. Directing mail across such gateways is generally straightforward. For example, to send mail from a CompuServe account to an Internet address, the CompuServe user simply adds the prefix ">INTERNET:" to the beginning of the recipient's Internet address, which is in the format described above. To send mail in the opposite direction, the Internet user converts the CompuServe user's e-mail address, which is typically of the form "XXXXX,XXXX" where X is a numeral between 0 and 9, to the Internet format "XXXXX.XXXX@ compuserve.com".

By using the Internet as an intermediary, you can often employ such conventions to send e-mail between two different host networks that are each connected to the Internet via a gateway (for example, between CompuServe and America Online). For more information about sending mail from one network to another, you can obtain the Inter-Network Mail Guide by using the URL: ftp://ftp.csd.uwm.edu/pub/ internetwork-mail-guide

You can also contact the administrator of your host computer for information on sending e-mail to other networks.

Structure of a Universal (or Uniform) Resource Locator (URL)

Just as individuals have e-mail addresses, host systems and resources within those hosts have addresses as well. A URL is an address of a resource available on the World Wide Web (WWW). These addresses consist of three components: the protocol used to interact with the resource, followed by "://"; the address of the host machine at which the resource is located, followed by "/"; and then the path to the resource in question. For the Inter-Network Mail Guide mentioned above, the protocol is "FTP"; the host machine is "ftp.csd.uwm.edu"; and the path to the resource in question is "pub/internetwork-mail-guide".

A growing number of navigational tools are able to interpret URLs and thus provide access to a document, a computer, a software program, or other resources on the Internet. Using a Web client such as Netscape, Mosaic, or Lynx makes it straightforward to open a URL, and use the resource of interest. When entering a URL into a navigation tool, be careful to enter it *exactly* as it appears in the source from which you obtained the URL. (Note that when using e-mail or URL addresses supplied in this book, the quotes should be omitted.)

Roadmap for the Internet

An excellent tutorial on navigating the Internet is called "Roadmap for the Information Superhighway Internet Training Workshop." This course has been archived and is available free of charge as a series of easily digestible "maps" (or "lessons") sent to the subscriber as e-mail messages that explain in understandable and practical terms how to use various functions available on the Internet (for example, listservers, gophers, WWW, and so on). To get the syllabus for the lessons, send an e-mail message to "listserv@ua1vm. ua.edu" that contains the following in the body of the message: "get map package f=mail".

A Sampling of Additional Medical Information Resources on the Internet

As discussed in Chapter 8, a growing number of medical information resources is available on the Internet. Access to these resources can be unpredictable during times when many people are trying to access the resource simultaneously or when the location of the resource has been changed. You should be aware that many Internet resources are "under construction" and that almost anyone can "publish" on the Internet. However, patience and care in accessing and using information available on the Internet is amply rewarded.

Below are several resources you may wish to try in addition to the ones mentioned in Chapter 8. (Note: Omit "URL:" when entering the URLs listed below into your browsing software, and enter URLs that appear on two lines as one continuous sequence.)

MEDICAL MATRIX. Database of clinical medicine resources on the Internet, categorized by disease and specialty.

URL: http://kuhttp.cc.ukans.edu/cwis/units/
medcntr/Lee/HOMEPAGE.HTML

NORTHWESTERN UNIVERSITY'S GALTER HEALTH SCIENCES LIBRARY SERVER. Contains links to various clinical resources, including Agency for Health Care Policy and Research (AHCPR) Practice Guidelines, the National Institutes of Health (NIH) Consensus Development statements, and others.

URL: http://www.ghsl.nwu.edu/

RURALNET. An evolving information system for rural physicians that contains files and bulletins from the Rural Information Center for Health Services as well as links to information from NIH, NLM, the World Health Organization, and more.

URL: http://ruralnet.mu.wvnet.edu

FAM-MED. An electronic conference and file area focusing on the use of information technology in family medicine. Includes resources such as software reviews, discussion archives, and a gopher server.

URL: gopher://ftp.gac.edu:70/11/pub/fam-med

HEALTH AND MEDICINE IN THE NEWS. Abstracts of health information published in the lay press.

URL: gopher://lenti.med.umn.edu:71/11/news

DIRECTORY OF MEDICINE-RELATED FAQs. This file is an evolving list of "frequently asked questions" documents on medicine-related topics posted to USENET newsgroups on the Internet. E-mail your request for a document to Bruce McKenzie:

brucem@cybertas.demon.co.uk

An Internet Working Group Focusing on Medicine

The exponential growth and rapid evolution of telecommunications in both the lay and medical area can make staying on top of current developments and useful resources a challenge. AMIA has formed an Internet Working Group that focuses on enhancing the use and utility of medical resources on the Internet. For additional information, contact AMIA (see under Introduction in this Appendix).

Publications

The number of publications of all types related to telecommunications has grown explosively along with popular interest in telecommunications. A sampling of articles, magazines, and books is provided below.

Medically Oriented Articles on Telecommunications

Anderson RK, ed. Symposium: the Internet connection. Bull Med Libr Assoc. 1994;82:391-433. A series of articles relating Internet resources and services to the needs of the health sciences community. A useful summary of Internet navigational programs is included.

Faughnan JG, Doukas DJ, Ebell MH, Fox GN. Cruising the information highway: online services and electronic mail for physicians and families. J Fam Pract. 1994;39:365-71.

Frisse ME, Kelly EA, Metcalfe ES. An Internet primer: resources and responsibilities. Acad Med. 1994;69: 20-4.

Glowniak JV, Bushway MK. Computer networks as a medical resource. Accessing and using the Internet. JAMA. 1994;271:1934-9. *See also* in the same issue: Lincoln TL. Traveling the new information highway, pp. 1955-6.

Kassirer JP. The next transformation in the delivery of health care. N Engl J Med. 1995;332:52-4.

Kleeberg P. Medical uses of the Internet. Journal of Medical Systems. 1993;17:363-6.

Internet and Online Services: General Reference Books and Other Sources

Braun E. The Internet Directory. New York: Fawcett Columbine; 1994.

Dvorak JC, Amis N, Feibel W. Dvorak's Guide to PC Connectivity. New York: Bantam Books; 1992.

Engst AC, Low CS, Simon M. Internet Starter Kit for Macintosh: Everything You Need To Get on the Internet (with disk). Indianapolis: Hayden Books; 1994.

Engst AC, Low CS, Simon M. Internet Starter Kit for Windows: Everything You Need To Get on the Internet (with disk). Indianapolis: Hayden Books; 1994.

Fraase M. The Mac Internet Tour Guide: Cruising the Internet the Easy Way (with disk). Chapel Hill, North Carolina: Ventana Press; 1994.

Fraase M. The Windows Internet Tour Guide: Cruising the Internet the Easy Way (with disk). Chapel Hill, North Carolina: Ventana Press; 1994.

Gilster P. The Internet Navigator. New York: John Wiley & Sons; 1994.

Kehoe BP. Zen and the Art of the Internet: A Beginner's Guide. 3d edition. Englewood Cliffs, New Jersey: Prentice Hall; 1994.

Krol E. The Whole Internet: User's Guide and Catalog. Sebastopol, California: O'Reilly & Associates, Inc.; 1992.

Lambert S, Howe W. Internet Basics: Your Online Access to the Global Electronic Superhighway. New York: Random House; 1993.

Online Access (monthly magazine) (800-366-6336).

PC World (magazine) (415-546-7722). The January 1995 issue is dedicated to the topic of connecting to the Internet.

Chapter 9. CD-ROM Technology and Full-Text Information Retrieval

Identifying Additional CD-ROM Products

As with telecommunications resources, the availability of medically oriented CD-ROM products is growing rapidly and in parallel with the expanding use of CD-ROM technology by the general public. Magazines devoted entirely to CD-ROM use can be found wherever magazines are sold, and popular computing magazines regularly contain feature articles on CD-ROM–related topics (*see*, for example, "50 Best CD-ROMs," *MacUser*, October 1994).

In the medical domain, some catalogs and directories are devoted entirely to CD-ROM products (for example, CMEA, Inc. [Continuing Medical Education Associates, Inc.], telephone: 800-227-CMEA or 312-733-0469; and *Interactive Healthcare CD-ROM Directory*, Stewart Publishing, telephone: 703-354-8155). Some general medical software catalogs (for example, Alpha Media, telephone: 800-832-1000) have entire sections devoted to CD-ROM products. A

chapter on CD-ROM in ACP's *Software for Internists* reviews several of the products discussed in Chapter 9, as well as several others.

Chapter 10. Portable Computing Devices

Identifying Medically Oriented Products and Information

Information on medical uses of portable computing devices is becoming more plentiful. Medical magazines are more frequently providing articles and vignettes about the clinical use of portable devices (for example, *see* "Tiny Computers a Big Hit in Medicine," *ACP Observer*, October 1994, p. 8).

Some general medical software catalogs (for example, *Medical Software Products*, telephone: 800-444-4570) feature separate listings for portable computer applications. In addition, device vendors are beginning to publish catalogs of medical applications available for their products. For example, Apple distributes *Newton in Healthcare: Solutions Guide*. Contact Apple representative Jane Curley at 714-222-2608 or send an e-mail to: Newton.Med@Applelink. Apple.Com

Online bulletin boards and listservers (*see* Chapter 8 and *see under* Chapter 8 in this Appendix) devoted to discussion of medical applications of portable devices are also growing in number. For example, anyone who can send and receive e-mail from the Internet can participate in the Newton Solutions in Medical Care discussion group. To join, send an e-mail to "listproc@dsg.harvard.edu" and include the following in the body of the message, "subscribe newtmed yourfirstname yourlastname". Similarly, AMIA's MedSIG forum on CompuServe has a section on clinical applications of portable computers.

Other Information Resources

As with telecommunications resources and CD-ROM programs, portable computing devices and applications are becoming increasingly popular with both the general public and the medical community. Magazines focusing on portable devices include:

The HP Palmtop Paper (bimonthly magazine). Telephone: 515-472-6330; fax 515-472-1879. The May-June 1994 issue focused on medical uses of the HP palmtop.

PC Laptop Computers (magazine). Telephone: 800-320-8522.

PDA Developers. A newsletter/journal on palmtop computing for the technically oriented. Contact Creative Digital Systems. Telephone: 415-621-4252.

Pen Computing Magazine. Telephone: 516-681-5208.

General-purpose computing magazines also periodically highlight portable devices. For example, *see PC/Computing*, January 1995 issue (800-365-2770), which is devoted to portable computing product reviews and reports.

Device developers can also be a useful source of information about their products. For example, Hewlett Packard supplies information about its portable products via a toll-free number (800-443-1254) as does Apple Computer, Inc., for the Newton (800-767-2775).

Many value-added online service providers have discussion groups devoted to hand-held computing devices. For example, CompuServe offers Go HP Handhelds and Go Palmtops, and America Online offers PDA forum.

Chapter 11. Computer Basics

The material presented in Chapter 11 should provide the background needed to successfully purchase and begin using computer hardware and software. As computers are becoming more of a natural appliance in everyday life, good information resources are becoming ubiquitous. Reviewing one or more popular computing magazines provides a quick overview of some of the "hot" products and topics. Similarly, calling for and reviewing a few free product catalogs provides an overview of available products, features, and prices. Once you have taken the plunge, various excellent books are available to help you get the most from your new hardware and software; be sure to check for current editions.

Mail-Order Catalogs for Hardware and Software

Global Computer Supplies: 800-845-6225

Mac Connection: 800-800-2222

The Mac Zone: 800-248-0800

Mac Warehouse: 800-255-6227

MacMall: 800-222-2808

Micro Warehouse: 800-367-7080

The PC Zone: 800-258-2088

Books about the PC

Davis F. The Windows 3.1 Bible. Berkeley, California: Peachpit Press; 1993.

Knorr E, ed. The PC Bible. Berkeley, California: Peachpit Press; 1993.

Magid L. The Little PC Book. Berkeley, California: Peachpit Press; 1993.

Murray K. Introduction to Personal Computers. 4th edition. Carmel, Indiana: Que Corporation; 1993.

Nelson KY. The Little Windows Book. Berkeley, California: Peachpit Press; 1992.

Books about the Macintosh

DiNucci D, Castro E, Abernathy A, et al. The Macintosh Bible. 5th edition. Berkeley, California: Peachpit Press; 1994.

Nelson K. Voodoo Mac. Chapel Hill, North Carolina: Ventana Press; 1993.

Que's Little Mac Book. Carmel, Indiana: Que Corporation; 1992.

Williams R. The Little Mac Book. 3d edition. Berkeley, California: Peachpit Press; 1993.

Index